BECOMING
PART OF THE RIBBON

Becoming Part of the Ribbon

MY PERSONAL JOURNEY

I hope you enjoy the book! Remember, Don't sweat the small stuff. Hugs, Sharon

Sharon S. Hart

Library of Congress Control Number: 2010904908
ISBN: Hardcover   978-1-4415-5566-3
                 Softcover   978-1-4415-5565-6

This book was printed in the United States of America.

To order additional copies of this book, contact:
Xlibris Corporation
1-888-795-4274
www.Xlibris.com
Orders@Xlibris.com
50364

CONTENTS

Acknowledgments

First of all, never would I have imagined that I, Sharon S. Hart, would be writing a book. I started writing these "updates" as a therapeutic way to get through my journey with breast cancer. It was you, my family and friends, that inspired me to turn my updates into a book. I know that this is not the best book that you have read, but my purpose is not to have it on the best seller list, rather, to have it as a remembrance of what I went through on my journey. It also serves to help others who have just heard the words "You have cancer" to be able to get through the battle. During the time of my diagnosis and treatment, as well as the writing of this book, I have many people that I would like to thank.

My husband, **Bill**, for making me feel so loved and beautiful every step of the way. You were always there to make sure that I was comfortable and safe. You have and still are fighting to understand why it had to be me, but I want you to know that we can't change what has happened, and we got through it. We are such a great team together, and we have proven to ourselves that we can make it through anything. I rely on you more than you know to be my best friend, husband, and supporter. I look forward to many years to come, and I don't ever want you to forget how thankful I am that we found each other. I love you with all of my heart!

William "Buddy", thank you for showing everyone that a real man or boy wears pink! You were so strong and helpful during the time of my treatments. Every time you came in to lay with me or check on me and then told me you loved me made me stronger every step of the way. I love you so much, and thank you for taking care of me when I needed it.

Zachary, thank you for giving me those waist hugs when we couldn't give the true hugs. I know that you may not remember much of what went on, but I hope that you will remember that we made it, and your love was more helpful than you know. I love you.

Also, thank you, Buddy and Zachary, for understanding why I couldn't play Wii with you while I was putting the book together. I have a lot of making up to do.

Mom and Dad, thank you for making me the person that I am. It is because of the two of you that I am as strong as I am. I may have made it look easy, but I wouldn't have been able to be this way if it wasn't for you. Mom, thank you for taking care of me before, during, and after my diagnosis. That motherly love is priceless and will never be lost. Thank you for being able to "have fun with it." Dad, thank you for being my chauffeur and for having those priceless moments that we shared talking, eating, cruising—and we can't forget shopping! I love you both so very much, and thank you again for everything that you have given me in my life. I couldn't have asked for better parents.

Joanne, thank you for being my emotional one. You were the one that worried for all of us, but regardless of the situation, you were always there for me. I will never forget how you helped Bill, Buddy, Zachary, and Darla during this time. I am so thankful for how close we are, not only in distance, but in friendship. I can't say enough, but thank you and I love you.

Brenda, thank you for being the hostess with the mostest! I think that this journey has made you and I understand each other better and made us closer. Your caretaking abilities are unspeakable. I will never forget how you welcomed me into your home and took such good care of me right after my surgery. You were my backbone in helping me understand so much and for watching over me during *all* of my surgeries. I thank you for getting me through some of my rough times and for being there for me. I love you!

John, thank you for just being you. You were the other half of the emotional one, which was helpful for both of you. Thank you for caring for me and for worrying about me. I hope that you can see that we did it and nothing can stop me from shoveling my driveway or driving your tractor. I love you and thank you.

Dave, thank you for fighting for our country. I know that you were not here during most of my journey, but I am very thankful that you are a part of our family. I am very proud of what you do and who you are. I love you.

Jessica and Jaylyn, I thank you for taking such good care of me during my journey. Your cards, flowers, kisses, and hugs were priceless. Jessica, it meant so much to me when you donated your hair at the Relay for Life.

You have such a big heart. Jaylyn, your concern for my boo-boos getting better made me stronger, and I thank you for loving me. I love you both very much.

Dr. Warren, thank you for being my guardian angel during this whole process. Your perseverance, calmness, and knowledge helped me get through the hard times that I had. We were able to get through it, and I wanted you to know how thankful I am for everything that you did for me.

To the rest of the **Dr.'s, nurses and staff** of the HGC, the Wilmington Hospital and the Arsht Surgi Center, I thank you all for taking such great care of me and for enjoying what you do. I appreciate all of the work that you did for me and nothing personal, but I hope that I do not have to see many of you again anytime soon!!

To the rest of my **family and friends**, thank you for reading my updates and being there for me. I can't personally thank everyone, but those of you that went that extra step know who you are, and I thank you.

I have learned many lessons along this journey, and I hope that I have expressed them to you. I hope that you enjoy every moment of every day of your life. Things can get tough, but you can work them out. Family and friends are so important to have, and I hope that you treasure every one of them. I hope that one day you will never have to hear the words "You have cancer." But if you do, I hope that you have a better understanding of what one can expect during the journey. Thank you again to all of you, and I am so thankful to be healthy and alive. I also am so very thankful to have the best family that anyone could ask for. Now go check your breasts and then give someone a hug!

Hugs to you,
Sharon

INTRODUCTION

It all started on the night of August 7, 2007, a Tuesday. I was at a Ladies' Auxiliary meeting at the firehouse where I volunteer, and on my way home, I felt a discomfort on my left breast. When I reached up, to my surprise, I felt a lump! When I got home, my sister Joanne was watching the kids, and I told her I felt a lump. I asked her if she felt something, and she thought she did also. We went into the bathroom, and I removed my shirt, and we checked again. The lump actually felt hard and like the size of a bouncy ball. I thought to myself, *I need to get this checked out.* I had the week off of work and had planned to go to a family fun center with our children the next day. My mom had found out about the lump, and she was instantly getting me to make a phone call to the doctor. I was planning on calling, but it was too late that day, and I would make the phone call the next day. I did not worry about it too much since I knew there was not too much I could do about it then. Also, not ever feeling a lump before, I was doubtful if that was what I was really feeling. My husband, Bill, was on night work; and I told him about the lump and that I was calling the doctor the next day.

Wednesday, August 8, 2007

When I got up in the morning, I planned to go to the family fun center with my kids Buddy (seven), Zachary (four), my nieces Jaylyn and Jessica, and their friends Nick and Haley. We all piled in the car and went. The kids had a blast. We got there at ten thirty in the morning and did not leave until two in the afternoon. By the time I returned home, I completely forgot about calling the doctor. I called my mom, and she asked if I called the doctor. "OOPS, I completely forgot."

Mom said, "Sharon, you better call right now." I told her that it isn't that I am not concerned, I just forgot. So I called my gynecologists, and learned that the office was closed. So I had to wait until tomorrow. I continued on with my normal activities. My sister Brenda, a registered nurse, called; and she said, "So what is this about a lump?" I told her that it was on my left breast, near my nipple (underarm side), and felt like the size of a golf ball.

"A GOLF BALL!" she said, and I replied, "OK, maybe a bouncy ball." She asked if it was hard, and I told her yes and quickly asked if that was a good thing. She said that it wasn't the best. Then I started thinking to myself that this may not be good. I told her I was calling the doctor tomorrow, and I would let her know.

Thursday, August 9, 2007

Tonight, I had planned a Longaberger® Hostess Appreciation Dessert night at my house for about nine to ten people. It would start at 6:30 p.m. I had some last-minute things to get ready, but I needed to call the doctor first. I called the doctor's office, but it does not open until 9:00 a.m., so I waited until then to call. I told the receptionist that I found a lump, and I needed to get it checked. She said the two doctors were not in today. The physician's assistant was in but was jam-packed. I asked her if it would take that long to get a lump checked. She put me on hold and then told me that I could come in, sit, and wait; but she could not guarantee me a time when I could see her. She also suggested that I call my family physician and see if they could see me sooner. So I called my family physician and learned that they do not open until 10:30 a.m. I then called my mom and filled her in, and we were both surprised about the doctors being so unaccommodating about something that can be so serious.

I got dressed and was getting ready to take Zachary to school. Joanne stopped by, and I filled her in. She was taking Jessica to school to see her new class and asked Buddy if he would like to go, and he did. I dropped Zachary off at school and drove to my family physician's office. I told them that I have found a lump on my breast and wanted to have it checked. The only appointment they had was at 2:00 p.m. I went ahead and scheduled the appointment and told them that if something comes up at my gynecologist sooner, I would take that appointment. I was surprised that they didn't just have me wait and check me sooner. I know that if this was serious, four hours would not make a difference on my prognosis. But mentally, it could have a huge impact. I left the office frustrated and headed for my gynecologist's office to sit and wait. I again called my mom and filled her in. I was not sure why I was doing it; she didn't need things like this to raise her blood pressure. Bill was at work, and I usually don't call him there unless I have to, but I felt the need to vent a little and fill him in on where I would be.

I headed to the Medical Arts Pavilion II, and while I was pulling in, my eyes were attracted by the sign that read Breast Center and Cancer Center. I was curious as to what the breast center was. As I was walking into the building, I asked the greeter (whom I have never seen before), "What is the breast center? Is this where they do breast exams, ultrasounds, and mammograms?" He answered yes, and I walked in the building. I walked past the breast center to get to my gynecologist's office. I don't think I ever really noticed that office before today. As I walked into my doctor's office, I found out that the receptionist is one of my patients (I am a Dental Hygienist). I let her know that I was told to come in and wait so the doctor could check the lump on my left breast. I told her that my family physician couldn't see me until 2:00 p.m., so I would take a chance there (it was then only 11:00 a.m.). I went and sat down, and my friend came over, and we caught up on things. The phone started ringing, and she stepped away. About fifteen minutes later, they called me back. I was thinking to myself, *Wow, that was a quick wait.* The nurse practitioner came in, introduced herself, and asked me a few questions—how and when did I find out about the lump, do I have a family history of breast cancer, etc. She asked me to remove my gown, but I did not tell her which breast I found the lump in. She did an exam on my breasts. I thought it was great because her mind was not focused in one area, and she was checking everything. She asked me to lean forward and let my breasts hang down. Then she had me sit up and raise my arms over my head. Then she had me lie on my back. She headed straight to the left breast and exactly where the lump was located. She felt around and said, "Oh, that is a good size." She measured it to be about four something. She felt that it was a cyst, but she wanted me to get an ultrasound to see if it was liquid or solid. If it was solid, she would remove it. If it was liquid, she could (1) drain it and hope that it doesn't return, (2) have me go through two menstrual cycles and see if it drains itself, or (3) I can't remember what the third option was. She said they might not be able to see the cyst with the ultrasound, so I didn't have to be alarmed. She gave me a script and told me to go to the Breast Center—imagine that. I thanked her for seeing me so quickly, and she told me that when she heard it was a lump, she took that as a priority and not to worry if it made her run behind schedule. I was glad to hear that. I got dressed and made a follow-up appointment after two months.

I walked down the hall to the breast center. As I walked in, there was a variety of people: old, young, with hair, no hair, walking, and people in wheelchairs. I went up to the desk, signed in, and sat down. They called me and asked if I had an appointment, and I told them that I did not, but my gynecologist sent me over. The receptionist checked with another staff person. They told me they could squeeze me in, but it would be about an-hour-and-a-half wait. I did not have any plans until tonight, so an hour and a half would be fine. I went back to the waiting room that had a TV and snacks. I told the receptionist that I had to make a phone call, and she said, "That's fine, but don't leave the building." She advised me to go to the hallway in case I could be seen sooner. I again called my mom and informed her about what was going on and asked her to call everyone else. I then called my family physician and cancelled my 2:00 p.m. appointment. I went back to the waiting room and got comfortable. I brought some reading materials, and they also had plenty of magazines. As I was sitting there, I noticed a room from across me and started to wonder what was going on in there. I saw an older lady go in there, and she still had her examination gown on. I thought to myself, *I wonder if she has breast cancer.* The other rooms were dressing rooms and treatment rooms (for mammograms and ultrasounds). The women about to have tests were in pink gowns.

I sat there for about an hour and a half, and they called my name. I went back, and they asked me to change into a gown, put my clothes in a locker, and take the key. When I was finished with these, the nurse was waiting, and she took me into a side room for the ultrasound. In the room, there was a technician and another lady dressed in business attire. She informed me that the machine was a new one, and they were familiarizing themselves with the buttons. The lady in business attire was training the staff on the new machine. I commented, "So I am the guinea pig, huh." They both laughed. I sat down, and they asked me to point to where I found the lump. I pointed to the lump, I lay down, and she marked my left breast. She put some gel on it and started the test. I certainly could not see what she was looking at, but she kept focusing on one area. She left the room and came back with a radiologist, who found an area that was questionable. He wanted me to get a mammogram.

We went to the next room to get the mammogram. That was my first one, and I was so curious I had to look at all the pictures and asked a whole lot of questions. My right breast looked good, but my left breast definitely had something going on in there. I think everyone assumes the worst when they are getting checked. After the mammogram, I got dressed, and the technician told me that the radiologist wanted to see me. I was thinking, *This can't be good since everyone else could just leave, and I had to see the radiologist.* I followed the technician into a darkroom. The radiologist and a nurse were there. The radiologist sat me down, showed me the area in question, and said that it appeared to be malignant. He introduced me to the nurse, and she explained what would follow. The radiologist then said, "You seem to have expected this to be malignant."

I said, "No, not really, but I am young, healthy, and I want to get this out of my body." He touched my leg and said, "You are going to be okay."

I then followed the nurse to the room that I earlier described. She thoroughly explained all the different biopsies that could be done and why they were performed. I was a little shaky, but I was just sitting there, taking it all in. She asked if I needed to call a family member. I told her that I would rather wait because I was more worried about how they would react versus what was being said. She informed me that there was a doctor available now if I wanted to do the core biopsy today. She spoke very highly of the doctor, so I trusted her opinion and went to visit the doctor, who was in the same office area. I did not have to worry about the time since my kids would be taken care of by my sister Joanne if I run late.

I was taken to another exam room, and while I was waiting, I felt the need to call my sister Brenda to get her opinion. But the doctor walked in so I hung up. She did her intro and said that she was going to do a core biopsy to see what was going on. She reviewed the film and told me that a nurse would be in for me shortly. It was already around a quarter past three in the afternoon, and I have not called any of my family yet. While waiting, I laid back and grabbed a magazine and tried to soak in the news. I felt as if I was numb or already accepting the news. I did not want to call anyone until I was done with all these procedures. The nurse came back in and reassured me that the doctor would take good care of me. I think she was surprised that I was taking all this so well. She stayed in there with me for a while and told me that I could call her anytime.

I was then taken to the procedure room. They asked many questions and had me mark an X on the breast that was getting the biopsy. There were two nurses in the room, and then the doctor came in. She numbed the area (not too painful) and made a small incision. I felt something cold run down my side, and why I thought it was saline and not my blood, I have no idea. While I was watching the ultrasound, the doctor took four core biopsies. She showed me the cores and gave me some instructions. The doctor told me she was putting a rush on the test, and she wanted to see me in her office on Monday. The nurse straightened everything up, and I thanked her immensely because she was the one who stayed late so this biopsy could be performed. The other nurse put a gauze pad on the incision area and wrapped the site with an Ace bandage. She gave me a prescription for Xanax and Vicodin and told me not to take a shower for three days. Did this lady know that it is the middle of August, and the temperature is about ninety-five degrees? While she was finishing her notes, she had noticed from my voice and my body that I was shaking, but I explained to her that it was just my nerves. I have also not had a chance to warm up since all the rooms were so cold because of the machines. She gave me a blanket and made sure I wasn't having an allergic reaction to the anesthesia. When I walked out of the room, the office lights were turned off. I thought to myself, *Oh my gosh, I closed the office. They really did stay late for me.* She walked me to the door and told me that I did a great job and wished me good luck with everything. It was almost five in the afternoon, and I was off to the day care to pick up Zachary. I was thinking that in an hour and a half, I would have ten ladies coming to my house. I would have to clean, set everything up, and tell my family about today. I should cancel, but I feel okay. But what if I feel pain, etc? On the way to the day care, I called Brenda and told her about the biopsy and that the doctors think the lump is malignant. She didn't know what to say, but I told her that I am okay with it. It is what it is, and I would have to wait until Monday to get the confirmation.

When I got to the day care, I saw my friend Michelle, who was invited to my house tonight. She didn't know if she would be able to make it tonight, and so she gave me some baskets that had to be given to Maggie, who was also invited. I told her that she did not have to worry about coming because I may not have the party, which was a Hostess Appreciation Night. She asked me if everything was all right, and I informed her that I would explain everything later but not to worry. She seemed puzzled, and later, I found out that she thought I was mad at her. When I picked up Zachary, I let him know that he had to be careful with Mommy because she has boo-boos on her boobies. When we got to the car, he wanted to watch TV, and I continued to think about canceling the party. The decision was final—I was canceling. I called Carla and let her know that I needed to cancel the party.

I explained to her that I had an unexpected procedure today and that I was not feeling up to having people over at the house. She asked, "Is everything OK?" I informed her that I would be all right and that I would fill her in later. She understood and hoped that I was okay and said that she would be thinking of me. We got home, and Buddy was at Aunt Doe Doe's (that is what they call my sister Joanne). Zachary walked down to her house. I called my mom to see if she was still coming over. She said that she was coming over, and she wanted to know what happened today. At that point, she still thought I was having the party. I thought I called everyone on the list who was expected to show up for the party.

Mom arrived, and we sat down to talk. I described the whole process. I told her that they took a biopsy, and it might be cancer. I was surprised that she didn't flip out, and then I thought, *Thank goodness for Xanax.* Don't get me wrong; she was in disbelief but looked like she was taking it well. During my talk with my mom, to my surprise, my nurse practitioner called to talk to me about the results. She said she was surprised with them but hoped that everything would go well. She went over a couple of other facts with me like the size of the lump and other things. I thanked her again for seeing me so rapidly and for the follow-up call. Next, the doorbell rang. It was my friend Cheryl. I forgot to call her and tell her that I was canceling. When she came in, I started filling her in. The doorbell rang again, and I couldn't think of who it could be. It was Maggie. Remember the one whom I was supposed to give the baskets to? (OOPS, forgot to call her also.) When she walked in, she had a look on her face that seemed to ask why the house wasn't set up for the party. I filled both Cheryl and Maggie in with what was going on. I continued to feel accepted and positive about my possible cancer. I was still second-guessing myself about canceling the party, but they reassured me that it was the right decision. I still went over with the two girls what I had prepared. We had some apple pie then called it a night. I felt bad about forgetting to call those two, but I was glad I could share this with them and see that they would be there for me if I needed them.

Buddy and Zachary came home from Aunt Doe Doe's, and I had to remind them to be careful of Mommy's boo-boos. I started feeling some discomfort, so I took some Tylenol since my prescriptions were not filled yet. My mom was about to leave, and I reassured her that everything would be all right. I told her to just have fun with me on this journey.

My sister Joanne (Aunt Doe Doe) is my emotional sister. I had told her earlier that they had found a spot, took a biopsy, and thought it could be malignant. She was in shock and very surprised about the news. She had the boys all evening, and hopefully, that would take her mind off of it.

Finally, I had called my husband Bill, on the way home from the testing center and told him the news. That night, he was getting off work at six in the evening and was going to his part-time job at the County 9-1-1 center. He asked if I wanted him to come directly home, but I had told him no since there was nothing that we could do about it right then. He said okay but ended up coming home anyway, which probably was a good idea since he handles emergency calls from the public, and his mind would be somewhere else. Please understand that I intentionally waited to tell Bill because I did not want him to worry. He still had hours of work, and I knew it would seem like forever if I told him sooner. I knew there was nothing we could do right then and that our lives were about to change.

We finally got the kids to bed and talked for a while tonight. I was trying to reassure him that everything would be all right. He has to work tomorrow, and I know it will be a tough day for him. But on Friday night, we have plans to go to the Blue Rocks baseball game with the Cub Scouts and sleep in a tent on the field after the game.

Friday, August 10, 2007

Buddy and I took Zachary to day care, and I informed his teachers Ms. Rose and Ms. Debbie of my possible cancer. I told them the same story about the testing and the results and that I am young and healthy and I can't change what is there. I can only do what needs to be done to get this out of my body. They were happy to see my spirits so high and wished me the best of luck. Buddy and I left the day care and came home to get ready for the game and sleepover. My mom called and wanted to know if I was still going to go to the game. Of course, she did not think it was a good idea for me to go. I told her that I was not dying and that I knew that if I was not feeling up to staying, then I would go to Brenda's to sleep after the game. When I told Brenda I might sleep over at her house, she got very excited. But I told her I would have to see how I felt. Bill got off work early and met us at the stadium. When we got to the game, it was cold. We were totally unprepared, not expecting this temperature in August. We went to the stadium store and spent $110 on sweatshirts. Oh well, it is just money, right? We had a great time at the game, but I could tell that Bill's mind was somewhere else. Jamie, the pack master, was talking to me about upcoming events and becoming a leader. He talked to me for about twenty minutes. Bill talked to Glenn (a friend from scouts) about becoming a co-den leader with us. We had not informed anyone of the news yet, so we played "normal" to everyone else. So finally, the game was over. We went to the car, got our camping gear, and headed out on the field. The boys were having a blast, running and playing football in the outfield with other scouts. I was feeling good but just a little tired. Bill seemed down and not as spirited as usual. They turned the lights out at midnight, and we tried to get a good night's sleep considering the I-95 traffic was right next to the stadium.

Saturday, August 11, 2007

Rise and shine time was at six in the morning, and we needed to be off the field by seven because the sprinkler system would come on. We packed up and went to get our breakfast. After breakfast, Bill headed back to work, and we headed home. Last night was fun, and I am glad we were there as a family. I came home and aired out all of our camping gear. I was feeling good, but the Ace bandage was starting to get itchy. I was counting down those three no-shower days. Thank goodness it has been cold. I can't wait until tomorrow to take this off and wash gently.

Anyway, Saturday night was our friend Scott's surprise fortieth birthday party. I arrived a little late, and Bill stayed home with the kids. He had to work on Sunday and did not want to go out for a drink. Everyone was glad to see me. I did not know who among them knew about the news, but I did not bring it up. This was Scott's party, and we could talk about everything at a later time. My mom, dad, and John (Joanne's husband) went home, and I stayed to be the designated driver for Joanne. As the party went on, I just sat back and observed as I felt a little self-conscious about my Ace bandage and the big bulge on my left side from the gauze. We left about half past twelve in the morning, and on the way home, Joanne and I got into a discussion. Of course, with alcohol come emotions, so when we pulled into her driveway, we had a nice talk, and she broke down. I comforted her and reassured her that it would be okay. She said to me that I was the one who was supposed to be crying, and she was supposed to be helping me. I told her that she was my emotional side, and that was okay. She was very worried and scared for me. Joanne and I are very close, and we tease all the time, saying we should move in with each other. We depend on each other for a lot of things, and I am so grateful that I have her as a sister and a friend.

Monday, August 13, 2007

Monday finally came—the big day for the results. The appointment was scheduled for 1:30 p.m. I worked at Dr. McAllister's that day until noon. When I got home, Bill told me that the office called and wanted us to come in early. We left right away and fought the I-95 traffic to get to the Wilmington office. When we went inside, the receptionist turned out to be my boss's niece, and Bill knows her husband through the fire service. I was a little anxious and had to go to the bathroom. But they called my name, and we went into the exam room. I put on my half gown and went to the bathroom. Bill already looked nervous. The doctor walked in, sat down with my charts, and started with a very detailed explanation. She confirmed that my lump was malignant and that it was something in situ, and due to this, the treatment would be a mastectomy. I just kept hearing in situ, in situ, in situ. She did not feel it was in the lymph nodes but could not confirm that until surgery. She said the cancer was in stage one, but I saw stage two on my charts. No worries though. I was all right with everything she was saying including the treatments. I just kept thinking, *Oh my gosh, I need to get my boob chopped off.* I looked over at Bill, and he was as white as a ghost, and his eyes were all red. I asked him if he was okay, and he just shook his head. The doctor continued and stated that she has set up my appointments: Tuesday—MRI, Wednesday—meet the plastic surgeon, and Thursday—multidisciplinary meeting at the Helen Graham Cancer Center. I was thinking to myself, *Hold on, I have to rearrange my whole schedule.* I then asked if there was a reason that we were doing this so quickly. "Is it that aggressive, or can we do this next week?" She said to me that breast cancer is slow-moving. *HAHA, I just had my yearly in February 2007, and it is only August 2007. I am getting a mastectomy. Slow-moving my ass.* Oh, sorry, back to what she was saying. If we wait one or two weeks, it will not make a difference. But here is the thing: we need to move quickly with younger people because of their lifestyles. Older people need more time to think about it. The longer I wait, the more I will think about it, ponder it, and worry about it. She could see that I am the type of person that does not like to inconvenience anyone. But now is when I need to make myself number one. I need to make my life as stress-free as possible for my immune system to be in top-notch condition. So with that said, I looked at her and said, "Nice, point well-taken." We will keep all the appointments and listen to her recommendations. She then said she would like to have surgery in about three weeks. Did I just hear her say three weeks? *Holy moly.* She said she would see us on Thursday at the Helen Graham Center and asked if I had any questions. As Bill was looking like he was ready to pass out, he looked at her and asked, "What is the prognosis, and is she going to make it?" The doctor reassured him that we caught it early, and I would be all right. She checked the biopsy site and said it looked good and that the surgi-strips would come off by themselves. I told her I was handling this well, but I was very concerned about Bill. She said that is to be expected and touched his shoulder and told him again that it would be okay. The nurse came in and gave us the appointment dates, locations, and a packet of papers to fill out for the Helen Graham Center.

When we got into the car, Bill and I discussed talking to Dr. H (my boss) about taking this week off. Of course, I was thinking that maybe I could just take a few hours off each day to attend my appointments. HELLO! Did I hear the doctor say not to stress myself out? What if the appointment runs late or my mind isn't into work? Okay, okay, it was two in the afternoon, and I knew my boss went out for lunch; and he normally goes home to eat. Bill called the office, and Pat told him that my boss just left for lunch. I called his wife, Julie, and asked if Dr. H was coming home for lunch. I told her that Bill and I needed to come by and talk to him.

She asked, "Should I be worried?"

I said, "No, I should be."

When we got there, his wife answered the door, gave us a hug, and invited us into the house. She told us to have a seat, and she would go get Dr. H. I asked how their vacation was, and she proceeded to tell us that minus the hospital visit, everything went well. While on vacation, he decided to start passing kidney stones, and the pain was excruciating. He came down walking in pain, sat down, and told us about his pain, the ambulance ride, and the hospital visit. When he was finished talking, I asked them if they knew why we were here. He didn't know, but Julie asked, "Are you pregnant?"

I said, "No, but I wish the news was that good." I then told them that I found a lump on my left breast, had a biopsy, and we just came from the doctor and confirmed that I have breast cancer. Both of them were speechless. Then Julie said, "Oh no, Sharon." With a smile on my face, I explained what I've been through in the last couple of days and what the doctor told me today. I then told them that I needed to have this week off due to the scheduled doctor's appointments. I said that I have tried to figure out how to work around the doctors' appointments, but I feel it is better if I just took off work. I was getting more nervous as the conversation continued.

I then said as I was beginning to cry, "I guess what I am asking is that I hope that you can support me in my decision and understand why I need to take off work." I then looked at Bill and said, "I can't believe I am crying in front of my boss, and I have been so strong with everyone else!" Julie told me that whatever I needed to do was fine, and they would figure out the schedule at work.

Dr. H said, "Well, here I am, sitting, complaining of pain with my kidney stone, and you have all this going on." He then said that we would get through this, and that he needed to head back to work. I asked him if he could tell the girls back at the office. We say our good-byes, and he asked us to keep them posted. When we left, it was three in the afternoon, and I told Bill that even though I asked Dr. H to tell the girls, we still had time to stop by the office so that I could tell them personally.

When we got there, Deb was leaving for lunch, but everyone else was there. I brought all the girls together and told them the news and the treatments needed. They were all in shock. Donna and Barb started to cry. (Bill later told me that he had to walk away because he felt a lump in his throat.) I went over and hugged them and reassured them that I would be okay. I would have a long journey ahead of me, but I was determined to win. I told them that I would not be in this week and that I would keep them updated. Auxi then walked in and instantly gave me a hug and said that she would pray for me. Dr. H returned, and I told him that I couldn't help myself that I felt I needed to talk with the girls personally. I informed the girls that I am very open about all this and asked them, in case any of my patients asks where I am, to please tell them what is going on. I also gave them my permission to give out my address and phone number if they asked. When we were leaving, they said to take care of myself and not to worry about the schedule—that it would be taken care of.

When we left Dr. H's office, we decided to go to Bill's part-time job at the County 9-1-1 center and let them know what was going on. Before we went there, we had to stop by and get Bill's truck from the dealer. They were doing some service work on it. We were then in two separate vehicles, but on the way to the county building, we talked on the phone with each other. When we got to the county building, we asked to talk with Bill's supervisor. We went to a conference room, and Bill told him that I was just diagnosed with breast cancer and that he would like to be taken off the schedule for the next two months until the surgery and all are over. His supervisor told him that this was not a problem and to let him know if there was anything that he or they could do for us. He shared with us that his sister is a breast cancer survivor and that there is light at the end of the tunnel. We were very appreciative that he was understanding and cooperative with our request. Then we left the conference room, and Bill took me on a tour of the new building. We stopped over and talked with Jamie (Michelle's husband). We filled him in and let him know that I was not mad at Michelle the other day. He informed me that we have been the topic of conversation at their dinner table, and he would be sure to fill Michelle in on the happenings. We had a lengthy conversation, and he then reminded us that his mother is a long-time breast cancer survivor. He told us to just let him know if they could do anything for us. I told him that Bill may need to talk with someone, and he said that he would have his father call him.

Bill then took me on a tour of the new 9-1-1 building. When we left, I called John (my brother-in-law, Joanne's husband) to see what he wanted for dinner. He said that we could cook some steak and others on the grill. We were having a family meeting tonight at Joanne's so that I could tell the whole family of the diagnosis.

On the way home, Bill wanted to stop at a convenience store for him to get a drink and for me to get some gas. I called Brenda to see if she was on her way down Joanne's house. And of course, through her questioning, I had to fill her in with the details. She had many questions, and I tried my best to answer them. What I was finding out was that when people explain things to me, I understand them. But when I explain things to people, they don't get it!

We all met down Joanne's house for dinner. With all the tension in the air, we all sat down and ate a nice dinner together. I was anxious (for lack of a better word) to have everyone finish eating so I could get it off my chest. After dinner, I told everyone that I would meet them all in the back room. We situated the kids and told them that the adults needed to have a meeting. I started off by telling everyone that my seminar was about to begin. I thanked everyone for attending this meeting. (I was trying to add some humor to it because I knew what was about to happen.) I then started by saying "Hello, my name is Sharon, and I have breast cancer." We got a little laugh out of it. I tried to explain to them everything that the doctor had told me, but everyone was a little confused. Questions were asked about the need for a mastectomy. Brenda then tried to explain in more detail. I told everyone that it was going to be okay and that we would all get through this. My dad asked some repetitive questions. He would never admit it, but I think it was more from fear or nerves. Bill asked Joanne if she was all right, and she responded, "HELL NO," and then she broke down, crying. We tried to get her to laugh, then I noticed that my mom had gotten up and went into Joanne's bedroom. I asked Bill if he would go see if she was all right. John was also taking it pretty hard. He informed me that during dinner, he choked on a piece of steak and said that it was due to his nerves. Bill and I said that we wanted to be very open with the kids. We wanted them to know what and why things would be a little different. We told everyone that I would go for my MRI tomorrow, and I would keep them all posted. We talked for a while and called it a night.

LET THE JOURNEY BEGIN.

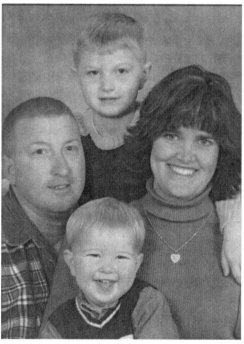

Family photo, 2007

Tuesday, August 14, 2007

After I had a good night's sleep, we planned the day for the kids, my MRI, and for Bill getting a nap before his night work. I called my friend Carla to see if she could watch the kids. I had told her about my diagnosis prior to this. She was more than happy to watch our boys for us. My appointment was at 12:00 p.m. at the Medical Arts Pavilion 1 next to the Christiana Hospital. While we were waiting to leave for my appointment, I had thought that this would be a good time to inform everyone of my diagnosis. I figured the best way to do this would be by e-mail, and this is how and why my journal began.

Hello Everyone,

I hope that everyone is having a great summer. I have some unfortunate news to tell you about myself. On Tuesday, August 9, 2007, I found a lump on my left breast; and on Thursday, I had it checked by the doctor through exam, ultrasound, mammogram, and finally biopsy (yes, all on the same day). I had my follow-up appointment yesterday, Monday, August 13, and the doctor confirmed that I have breast cancer. Everything is moving very quickly for me and my family, but we are holding up very well. I have accepted that I have this dreaded disease, but I can't take it away by becoming depressed that I have this. I have a very positive attitude, and I will get "IT" before "IT" gets me. I have several appointments this week with doctors and at the Helen Graham Center. The doctor has recommended the treatment to be a mastectomy, and we will not know if I will need radiation or chemotherapy until after the surgery. The reason for the mastectomy versus lumpectomy or trying chemo/radiation is that the site is small, but I have a large area of "scattered" malignancies that she feels we may not get just by doing lumpectomy/chemo/radiation. She does not feel that the lymph nodes are involved, so keep your prayers on that thought. I may have the date of the surgery on Thursday, and she noted that it may happen in as early as the next three weeks.

I would like to carry on my life as if this disease is not in my body. As most of you know, I like to keep busy with my boys' baseball and Cub Scouts and Ladies' Auxiliary and Longaberger®, but I do not know what to expect. I just ask for your support in this time of my life. Don't be afraid to call and ask me for something. If I can't help you out, I will let you know. Please keep in contact with me as you normally would and try not to worry about me. I will keep you informed of my progress. I have a lot of support from my family and friends, and I know that I will make it. Please keep me in your prayers, and after you read this note, GO CHECK YOUR BREASTS!

It was time to start the day. We dropped the kids off at Carla's and asked if Zachary could stay versus go to preschool, more out of convenience for us. She was fine with that, and off we went. When we got to the office, we went to the receptionist to check in. They had some paperwork for me to verify. After carefully checking it out, I did find some grammatical mistakes on their forms, and I brought it to their attention. Bill gave me a hard time (jokingly, of course). As I was sitting there, I kept telling myself that the MRI was mind over matter, but I was still a little nervous. When they called me back, they told Bill that it would be finished in about an hour and asked if he wanted to leave and come back. I gave him a kiss, and off I went.

When I got back to the changing room, the nurse asked me to change into a gown, put my clothes in a locker, and take the key (sounds familiar). As I was getting undressed from the waist up and removing all my jewelry, I noticed a list of music that I could listen to during the procedure. I thought, *Great, that would help me get through this.* I left the changing room and waited in the hallway. The nurse returned and took me to the MRI room. She asked me to have a seat on the machine, and then she explained the process and said that it would take thirty minutes. She also told me that she needed to place an IV so that they could use it for the dye to show the pictures. I informed her that starting an IV on me is tough, and she went and got someone who was very good at starting IVs. She looked at the left arm, nothing there. She went to the right arm, nothing there. Then she went to my left hand. She found a vein she could work with, and off we went to the next step. I asked for the nurse to come back in, and I asked her about the music. She informed me that there was music, but I wouldn't be able to hear it. OH CRAP! She told me that when she places me in the MRI machine, she would be stepping out of the room. She gave me a buzzer to hit in case I needed her, but she told me not to use it as a panic button. She also told me that when the machine turns on, it would sound like a jackhammer. This sound would last about ten minutes. I thought to myself, *I do not like this very much.* She asked if I was ready. "I guess so," I said. She put me in the tube, and oh crap, when I looked up, all I could see was a white tube with a blue stripe going down the center. This was not cool. I hated it already. She said that she was leaving the room. I heard the metal door shut, and my anxiety level began to rise. I thought that I could not do it, so I hit the "panic button." She asked if everything was all right. I told her that I needed to be pulled out of the tube for a minute. I heard the metal door open, and I was pulled out of the tube. *Whew, this is going to be a lot tougher than I thought.* I just kept thinking that I was only in a tanning bed—NOT. She asked me if I would like something over my eyes, and I said, "Sure, let me try that." She grabbed a towel and put it over my eyes. I told her that that would be better, so she put me back in the tube and left the room. Over the intercom, she asked if I was all right. I told her that I was okay, and she said we were about ready to begin. All of a sudden, I heard this noise. It was like a jackhammer, and then the sound would change slightly, but still like a jackhammer. I was lying in the tube, trying to think of a nice, relaxing place. I began to think about being at the beach since my friend Chrissy and I were going there on Sunday. Oh heck, that wasn't working either. I was lying in an enclosed tube, and I started feeling claustrophobic. Okay, relax, take a deep breath. Remember, mind over matter. It will only be a little while longer. I took a deep breath and felt them getting louder and shorter. I think I was ready to hyperventilate! A little while longer, the jackhammer stopped. The only sound after that was my beating heart. Finally, she asked, "Are you OK?"

I said, "Yes." Then the door opened, and she slid me out. WOW! That was much harder than I thought. She told me that I did a good job. I got up and went to sit in the chair that was in the room. I told her that it was much harder than I thought. She said that in the next part, I would be on my stomach, and it would take about twenty minutes. "TWENTY MINUTES," I said. I told her that I felt nauseated. She offered me a drink of water, and I refused. I refused because I would probably have to pee halfway through the next portion of the test. She asked me if I wanted her to get Bill, and I said no because he was running some errands. I went over to the table, and she told me to take my time. I apologized because at that time I wanted that drink of water. I took a small sip and said, "Let's do this." I laid on my stomach and put my boobs between some slots so they could hang down. She said to position myself so that I was comfortable. She explained that this was the longer test. There would be a few different sessions, the noise would turn off, and the dye would be pushed into the IV. I got excited because I thought she would come back in and administer the dye, but she told me it would be pushed in the IV by a remote control. I asked, "How is that possible?"

"Look through the tube, do you see that coil tube?" she asked. "That will get hooked to you prior to starting this test." I apologized for asking so many questions, but I liked to know the specifics. She told me to ask as many questions as I needed to. She then started to slide me into the tube.

Once inside the tube, I could see the other side of the "tunnel," and it was open. YEAH! I told her this would be much better since I could see outside the tunnel. I got comfortable and asked if I could have a pillow, and she said sure. Before she left the room, I asked her if we could try the radio. I knew that I wouldn't be able to hear it that well, but it may take my mind off of where I was and help me concentrate more on what was on the radio. I got comfy, and then I heard the metal door close again. Over the intercom, she asked if I was ready and turned on the radio. I thought to myself that this was going to be all right. There went the jackhammer sound again, but I concentrated on hearing the music. Believe it or not, I think I was so relaxed that I fell asleep. The machine turned off, and the nurse asked how I was doing. I said, "Fine, the music is helping." She said she was going to start the dye and that the next series would take about six minutes. It started, and anytime I got nervous, I opened my eyes, saw the opening, and relaxed again. Before I knew it, it was done. It got very quiet in the room, and then I heard the metal door open. She slid me out; I sat up and said, "YES, I did it!" I would definitely say that lying on my stomach was better than lying on my back. She walked me back to the dressing room and told me that the results would be completed in a few days.

I changed, put on my jewelry, and was looking forward to seeing Bill. As I opened the door, there he was, waiting for me with a smile on his face. I told him about the whole experience. He told me that he went to Home Depot to pick up some things and to the drug store to pick up some Benadryl for Buddy. (He had some small bumps on his back, and this usually does the trick.) We headed back to Carla's to pick up the kids. She said they had a great time and were good listeners. We headed home, and Bill went to get a short nap before going to night work. It is going to be a tough week for him, but he is determined to make all my appointments. Bill is still in shock about the news, but has not expressed his feelings with me yet. I will continue to work on that.

Later, I decided to check and see if I had received any responses from my e-mail, and WOW, was I ever surprised. I had pages of inspirational messages from my friends. This was when I knew that it was a good idea that I decided to keep a journal of my experience with my cancer. It felt therapeutic writing and reading the comments. So the rest of this journal is actually what I wrote during my journey.

Wednesday, August 15, 2007

Bill got home from work around seven in the morning and helped me get the kids ready for child care. After we dropped them off, we headed toward our next appointment. This appointment was with Dr. B, the plastic surgeon. We had a little trouble finding the office, but we made it on time. When we walked in, we noticed how nice the office was. We checked in with the receptionist and took a seat. Just a few minutes later, we were called back to the room. Dr. B was a very nice lady. She sat down and talked with us for a few minutes. She explained the choices for reconstruction.

1) Implants—less recovery time (two to four weeks), realistic-looking, and if need be, we could do a lift on the other side to make them "match"
2) Abdominal Tram Flap—longer recovery time (four to eight weeks), more invasive. It is done by tunneling the fat from the stomach up into the breast. More realistic-looking and feeling. She could do a lift on the other side to make them match. There is also a risk of getting a hernia or blood clot which might end up in failure.
3) Dorsal Flap—similar to above, but it takes tissues from the back and tunnels it into the breast. I am not too interested in this option, and she felt that it was not one for me either.

After all the explanations, I was heading more for the abdominal tram flap. I could get new boobs and a tummy tuck at the same time. My thought was that it would give a more realistic look and feel. I was not looking forward to the recovery period, but what is a girl to do? She left the room and asked me to get into a gown so she could examine me. While she was out of the office, Bill and I discussed some things and looked at my breasts, wondering what they would look like when this was all finished.

She returned to the room and looked at my stomach and told me that I had enough fat to do the tram. We could also lift the other breast to make them symmetrical. She showed us pictures of her work for both the implants and the tram procedure. They were very odd-looking without the nipples and areolas. She then explained to Bill (because he asked how they do it) how a nipple could be made and that it would stay erect all the time. I think Bill liked this idea. She talked for a little longer, explaining everything to us. She asked if we had any questions. We did not have any, but I did inform her that I was going to get a second opinion. She strongly agreed to that and told me that if there was ever a doctor who did not agree to that, she would encourage us not to see them. She said good luck to us, and we proceeded to the front desk. I honestly cannot remember the rest of the day, but I do know that it was a tough decision.

Thursday, August 16, 2007

The kids and I woke up, and Bill came home from work. We took Buddy to Aunt Doe Doe's and Zachary to preschool. We met Brenda at "The Pathway of Hope," also known as the Helen Graham Center, for our multidisciplinary meeting. Once I checked in, they asked me to come back by myself so they could get my vitals. A nurse, Nancy, got my vitals, gave me some information in a bag, and asked if I had received my notebook. I told her that I had not, and she told me that she was going to go get one and be right back. Well, she wasn't kidding about a notebook because it was a three-ring binder filled with information. It was a little overwhelming. Next came the psychologist, who looked like she was about twelve years old. She had a short discussion with me because two doctors walked in. They said hello and started talking to each other while looking at my information. They washed their hands and continued talking about me. I jokingly said, "I am sitting right here, and I can hear you!" They apologized, introduced themselves as Dr. W. and Dr. Strasser and asked me a few questions. They informed me that they were going to examine me, and afterwards, we would all meet in the other room. After they had left, Nancy informed me that they were double-booked today and apologized again for their actions. She asked me to get dressed, and then she took me to the meeting room where Bill and Brenda were waiting for me. We waited a little while, and they informed me that they were waiting for one of the doctors. Then the door opened, and in walked Dr. D, Nancy, the psychologist, Dr. Strasser, and Dr. W. Talk about intimidating. The meeting began with Dr. D reviewing that the good news was that the right breast looked clear—no sign of malignancy. Dr. W told me to stop taking my birth control pills immediately due to the positive estrogen receptor and that most likely, chemotherapy would be needed due to the fact the cancer was invasive. With that, Brenda was taken aback. This was something she did not expect to hear, and I took it to be more serious than what I thought. The actual diagnosis was called invasive ductal carcinoma in situ (DCIS for short). Dr. Strasser stated that he was unsure at that time if radiation would be needed.

Now, this was where the curve ball came into play. Dr. D noted that due to my age and since the only family history of breast cancer was my mom-mom at age 83, she would suggest that I do some genetic testing. This would let me know if I carry the BRCA I (breast cancer I) or BRCA II (breast cancer II) cancer gene. If I have either gene, that would mean that I have a sixty-two percent chance of getting cancer in the other breast and a higher risk for ovarian cancer. It would also mean that my sisters have a forty percent chance of getting breast cancer. At that point, I was shocked and felt a little uneasy. The decision that I thought I had made about the reconstruction was then in question. Dr. Strasser and Dr. W excused themselves due to the other consultations they had to get to. As Dr. D continued to talk with us and Brenda and Bill were asking questions, I began to get confused and overwhelmed with the information that was just given to me. I calmed down, and she asked me if I wanted to meet with the genetic counselor. I told her yes. She went to get it set up and told me that it was going to be okay. I asked her when we would get started because I was getting a second opinion with a plastic surgeon today. She seemed a little taken back when I mentioned this (I should have remembered what Dr. B had said about doctors who weren't for getting a second opinion). Anyway, she told me that until I decide on the plastic surgeon, we could not schedule anything. The meeting was over, and we went into the next room where the genetic counselor was waiting. By this point, I have calmed down. She apologized for it being done so quickly and hoped that it was not too overwhelming. She got started by explaining what genetic testing was, and she wanted to know if I wanted to go ahead with it. I said yes, and she began by asking me questions pertaining to my family history. She explained that they would get a blood test, and it would tell me if I carry the BRCA I or BRCA II gene. The test results would not return for thirty days, which meant it wouldn't be back prior to my surgery. She further explained that if it was positive, I would have a higher risk for ovarian cancer. The test would cost $3,158, and if it is positive, then my family could be tested, and it would cost them $350. Gee, they get a good deal. No fair! I asked her that if there is a test to find this gene, then why isn't it done on most people for prevention. Answer: Because insurance won't cover it unless you have been diagnosed. Go figure!

We were unable to get the test done that day, but we would schedule it before we leave. We were dismissed, and Bill left so he could get some shuteye before night work.

I went with Brenda since my second opinion was later on that day, and she was going with me. (Bill was disappointed that he couldn't make it, but was glad that I wouldn't be by myself.) We drove into Wilmington to get some tax information complete for Dave (Brenda's hubby) while he was in Iraq. When she was finished, we went to Houlihan's for lunch. She said that she would buy me lunch since I had cancer. Of course, she said that jokingly. You have to have some humor about this whole ordeal. Lunch was yummy, and then we headed over to Dr. Warren's office for the second opinion. The office was right across from the HGC, very convenient. After the paperwork, we were asked to go back, and when she came in, I automatically noticed this calmness about her, not to mention her good sense of style. She explained a little more and let me see the expander and feel the implants. I never thought that I would be shopping for boobs! We did discuss the possibility of a double mastectomy. She stated that it could be done as a preventative and that it would strictly be my decision, but I didn't have to decide right that second. Dr. Warren also suggested that if I'm not thinking of having anymore children, then Bill should go for the snippy snip. My life was being dictated as I went on. I am very thankful to have two healthy boys and am okay with this recommendation. I felt comfortable with her and was glad that I went for the second opinion. Not only did I choose Dr. Warren due to the calmness that I felt in her but also due to her convenient location. I informed her that I would like her to be my plastic surgeon, and she stated that she would call Dr. D and set up a time for surgery. Someone would call and let me know of the details. On the way home, I thanked Brenda so much for being there to support me, knowing what questions to ask, and recommending Dr. Warren.

That night, I had a long thought and discussion with myself and family, and my final decision was going to be a double mastectomy with reconstruction being implants. Even though my test results from the gene testing would not be available prior to surgery, I still want to go with the double. I do not want to take the chance of me having the gene and then possibly having to go through this again. I also feel that if I only have one breast, then I will constantly be comparing the real one with the fake one. So why not make them equal and make them both fake? Another thing is that I will always be perky in the chest area, and who knows, I may not have to wear a bra. See, there are good things that can come from everything. The reason that I am not going for the tram is that I have learned that I do not have the best of luck, and once you tell me that there could be failure due to a blood clot or you can get a hernia, that is all you need to say. Imagine going through all of that recovery just to have failure, and from what I hear, it really isn't a tummy tuck that you get anyway. I am comfortable with my decision, and my family backs me one hundred percent.

Friday, August 17, 2007

I worked half-day at Dr. McAllister's, and then Brenda, Joanne, the kids, and I headed down to Chincoteague for the weekend. Brenda has a trailer down there, and it is very relaxing, just what I need. We had a great time, and I pretty much laid back not only because I wanted to but because my sisters were making me. I had some moments when I was getting my bathing suit on, thinking how different I was going to look and that these saggy things would be gone soon. Oh well, let's put on some sunscreen, and go to the beach. You know, that is another thing. Will I think differently about the sun and not stay directly in it? Probably not, but I will be more conscious of it. Here is a thought, remember lying out in the sun and putting baby oil on! At least we don't do that anymore.

Bill was going to Pittsburgh on a bus trip with a friend of his to see the Phillies play. He checked in with me frequently to make sure I was doing okay. I reassured him all was well and I was relaxing.

Wednesday, August. 22, 2007

Today is Buddy's first day of school, and he is going into second grade. He seems to enjoy school. We are excited to have a teacher who actually taught Bill when he was in elementary school. Last night, we had a walk-through at the school so that he would know where to go, and we also informed Ms. Phillips about my upcoming surgery and treatments. She seemed very understanding and that she would "look after" Buddy.

I dropped Zachary off at preschool and headed for my pre-op appointment with Dr. Warren. Bill was unable to make this appointment due to work. He couldn't stand that he wouldn't be there, but I informed him that this was going to be a quick preview to get the date of the surgery. I wanted him to keep his vacation time for when I might need him more. He reluctantly agreed and went to work. The appointment with Warren was just that. She checked to see what my final decision was going to be for the reconstruction and if I had further questions. She reviewed with me that the surgery would take about four hours and that Dr. D would do her part first and then she would place the expanders after, but that she would be there for the whole surgery. This made me feel good. The date of surgery would be on Friday, September 14, 2007, at 9:30 a.m. with the surgery starting at 11:30 a.m. She has been able to schedule it at the Wilmington Hospital, and I was glad because Brenda works at the surgicenter right next to that, and she knows some of the nurses there. Dr. Warren took me to the surgical scheduling coordinator, and she reviewed paperwork and times with me. She didn't seem to be a very friendly person. It is amazing what a little eye contact and a smile can do for a person, but I guess not today.

When I left, I called Bill to fill him in on the details and then called the rest of my family. My cell phone is going to get some use these upcoming months.

Saturday, August 25, 2007

Today is Buddy's birthday party. He will be turning eight on August 31. We decided to have a "carnival"-style party for him which included a dunk tank, beanbag throw, water balloon fights, and Italian water ice. It was pretty warm that day, but everyone had a great time. It also felt like a celebration before the big surgery.

I have felt great and have gone on living as if it was like any other day. I plan on working up to the day before my surgery and going about my business like usual. I can see my family worrying about me, but I keep reassuring them that it is going to be okay.

Sunday, August 26, 2007

My day at the beach with my longtime friend Chrissy is finally here. I had not filled her in on my diagnosis yet. I purposely did this so that we could talk about it face-to-face. The funny thing was that prior to leaving, she asked if I could drive because she wasn't feeling up to it. Not hesitating, I said yes but asked her what was going on. She sort of smiled, and I instantly guessed that she was pregnant! She confirmed my guess, but I was still in shock about her news. This was going to be her third child, but it was unplanned, and we all know how that financial concern comes over all of us. We had a great conversation about the pregnancy, and I was thinking, *Wow, how do I bring up my diagnosis without putting a damper on this great news?* There really was no way to do it so I just had to come out and tell her. She felt so bad for not being too happy about her pregnancy when I was sitting there with cancer. I told her not to feel bad and I would have done the same thing. We talked all day and comforted each other with our upcoming events. I can't express enough how important it is to have friends whom you can lean on. Chrissy and I don't talk every day, but when we do, it feels like we haven't skipped a beat. I am very lucky to have a number of friends like her. We ended our day and agreed to try and continue our tradition by going to the beach, kid-free, for the day.

Thursday, August 30, 2007

I have my appointment for my blood work for the genetic testing. I went to the HGC, and the nurse was great with finding my vein. She packaged up the sample, and now the wait begins. The results will not be back for thirty days.

Friday, August 31, 2007

Today is Buddy's actual birthday, and since he has school, I brought cupcakes to school for his classmates to enjoy. We also had family come over tonight for the opening of more gifts. We try to do a friends' party and then a family party. The family party is usually on the actual birthday. So, here was a day when cancer was not the topic of conversation. It was the day for my Budman!

My Update

Monday, September 10, 2007

The last week has been pretty uneventful. I have been going about my business like normal. I received a phone call from the nurse who would preregister me for my surgery. I guess it's not really a dream. I have a pre-op appointment with Dr. D at 3:30 p.m. I plan on going to this by myself for the same reason as going alone to Dr. Warren. It should be pretty simple.

I went to the breast center, where one of her offices is located, and I waited to be called back. I ran into the nurse who saw me at the initial diagnosis, and she asked how I have been doing. I filled her in and told her when my surgery is. She wished me luck and said she would see me again. Dr. D. walked in. She reviewed my X-rays and informed me that the unanswered questions are still if the lymph nodes are affected and if and how much chemo/radiation I may need. The lymph nodes are tested at surgery and more in depth afterwards. This would determine the amount of chemo/radiation. I personally would like to have chemo as a preventative even if the nodes are not affected. I will not know the official results for seven to ten days after surgery, which by the way she informs me that I will be in the hospital for 23 hours! You might think I was just getting my tonsils out. We discussed what I have decided as far as surgery was concerned. I filled her in on my choice to get a double mastectomy, and she seemed okay with it. She has such a motherly feel about her, and when I left, I felt confident and as if she was proud of me. The appointment seemed rather quick, and she said she would see me on the fourteenth.

Later that night, the phone rang, and it was Dr. D! To my surprise, she was calling me in regard to my decision to have a double mastectomy versus a single one. She went on to tell me that she was looking over my chart, and she felt that my decision was very aggressive. *What!* I thought to myself. *I just left her office about three hours ago. Why is she calling to question my decision now?* She asked me why or how I made my choice, and I informed her of the reasons: (1) I was unsure if I had the gene, and I didn't want to take the chance; (2) If I did get it in the other breast, I wouldn't want to have to go through this again; and (3) It would be easier for me not to compare the fake versus the real. She told me that I have a very healthy breast on the right side, and if I was to get cancer later on, then we would just do the same process. Wasn't that just one of the reasons I wanted to do both now? I was pretty confident about my decision and was a little upset that she just saw me and did not bring up any of these concerns or questions during my appointment. My surgery date was in four days, and I have gone from feeling confident about my surgeon and thinking that she was proud of me to thinking that she was questioning my decision and wondering if I should have this surgeon work on me. We ended the conversation, and I instantly called Brenda and filled her in on what just happened. She was very upset about Dr. D's professionalism, and we talked for a very long time. She reassured me that I have made the right decision and that I have to make sure that I was comfortable with her doing the surgery. I put the kids to bed, called Bill, and filled him in on what had just transpired. He wished that he could be home to comfort me, but I reassured him that I would be okay. As I lay in bed, I tried and figure out the reason for the phone call. People who know me know that I try to look at the good side in most things. I came to the conclusion that maybe she was doing it to make me second-guess myself and make sure that it was the right decision for me. Sounds good, right? If this was the case, I was not sure that I would go about it in that matter. Anyway, it gave me a sense of calmness, and I was able to go to sleep.

The next couple of days, I discussed it with coworkers and some of my patients, which, I must say, being a dental hygienist, is almost like going to a psychiatrist. I let out all of my feelings, and my patients give me advice. During this whole time, I was still unsure as to why this doctor was doing this to me. I had also spoken with other breast cancer survivors, and it seemed that I did know what I wanted and that she couldn't change my mind.

Wednesday, September 12, 2007

I had a home show to do at my friend Amy's house, and as I was driving home, I saw a number on my phone that I didn't recognize. I played the message, and it was Dr. D calling, wanting me to call her back. When I got home, Bill told me that Dr. D called and wanted me to call her. Wow, she must really have to talk to me. I went into my bedroom and gave her a call at her home. She basically wanted to apologize for making me feel the way that I did. She still felt that it was an aggressive decision but understood that it was my decision. I told her how she upset me by questioning my decision and for doing it four days prior to surgery. I got pretty upset while talking to her, and she could tell. I did appreciate the call, and it made me feel a little more confident about her doing the surgery. Of course, I filled Bill in on our conversation and called Brenda to let her know what happened. Then off to bed we went.

Thursday, September 13, 2007

Today was my last day at work. It is hard to believe that just five weeks ago, my life took such a turn for the worse. I am planning on taking at least four weeks off, and who knows after that. My patients and coworkers have been very supportive during this first part of my journey. I left by giving them all hugs and telling them that I would keep them informed with my journal.

Brenda offered to have me stay with her for a couple of days after the surgery. This is what she sent me in an e-mail:

> *"I was thinking that when you come home on Saturday, I would love to take care of you for a couple of days. I don't know if you would want to stay here for a night or two. At least until you got yourself squared away and you have figured out what will be going on with things like the drains and dressings, etc. I thought it might be easier without the kids. I know that you like them to be involved, but it might be a good idea to get a routine down before you involve them. Just thought I would throw it out there, and you let me know. I have a really comfy couch and bed. I'll even get you ice cream if you are good.*

> *Love you,*
> *Brenda*

I let her know that I was going to take her up on her offer, and I looked forward to our time together.

As part of my update I added this to my e-mail:

I have been helping my hubby, sister Joanne, and my mom get through this. They are doing much better as they and we talk about it. As you can see, I am very open about the process and am not ashamed or embarrassed, if that is the right word, about my breast cancer. I have been amazed on the outpouring of support from my friends and family. I thank all of you for that, and I will continue to keep you updated. We went and bought a laptop so that I can keep busy while I am recuperating.

Anyway, the countdown is on, and I am ready to take the challenge and win! Thank you again for all of your thoughts and prayers and reassurance. Once again, if you have not had your mammogram, then do it now.

I will talk to you soon, and have a beautiful day

Sharon

After Bill and I got the kids to bed, we decided to have a little photo session of my breasts. We took pictures of me standing up and with me having them hang down. I don't tell you this to gross you out but to tell you how much it showed me. I could not see the abnormality before, but when we were looking at the pictures, it amazed me how deformed my left breast really was. If you really want to see what your breasts look like, have your significant other take a picture. Not only will it give you a true view of what you look like, but your significant other will enjoy it as well. Needless to say, we had a very nice night together.

Friday, September 14, 2007

The day has arrived. We got the boys ready for school and reminded them that Mommy would be in the hospital when they get home today. They gave me big hugs, told me that they love me, and wanted to know if they could call me tonight. I reassured them that they would be able to talk to me, and I would miss them very much while I am gone. Kids are so strong with this sort of thing; it was just like any other day. Buddy got on the bus, and we took Zachary to preschool. The teachers knew that today is the day and wished me luck and asked Bill to call them with an update.

We headed to the Wilmington hospital, and I was feeling okay. We parked and started walking up to the entrance, and of course, with Bill's and my sense of humor, I told him to just think that I was walking in with two boobs, and when I leave, I will have none! We giggled and knew that we would get through this together. I got to the floor where my surgery would be and went to register. While you are sitting there, you always wonder what everyone is getting done. Joanne and my mom were planning on sitting with Bill while I was in surgery. They were meeting us there.

They called my name after a short wait, and I went back to get my vitals taken. The nurse asked me all sorts of questions, and one of them was "Are you pregnant, or is there a possibility that you could be?" I would hope not, but there was always that possibility. She said we would be safe and have me take a test. A heated rush came over me. I was thinking, *What if I was pregnant?* That was all I needed to add to my adventure. Luckily, the test came out negative, and we moved on to more questions and needle pricks. I finally got into my beautiful gown, hair cap, and booties. They told me that they would go and get Bill and that I would be going back shortly. When Bill came back, he told me that my mom and Joanne are caught in traffic and weren't there yet. My mom was frantic because she didn't think she was going to see me before I go back, but I talked to her on the phone and told her that I would be fine and she would see me smiling after my surgery. Brenda showed up, and they told me that it was time to go to back. Bill gave me a hug and a kiss and told me he loves me. I did the same, and off we went. We walked down this hall and out a door to another hall. To my surprise, it was the hall where we went to register and Bill was there, waving, watching me go through the doors. It probably sounds bad reading this, but to me, it wasn't too bad because they had to take my glasses from me, and I was practically blind so I could not see what his facial expression was.

Once I was in the pre-op "holding room," Brenda introduced me to the nurses, anesthesiologist, etc. I was in my happy mode and told them that if I run into them again, I wouldn't recognize them because unless they come right up to my face, I couldn't see them. They got a laugh at that and couldn't get over how much Brenda and I sound a like. They got me hooked up. They had been forewarned about my veins, but they did awesome. As I was waiting, Brenda asked permission for my mom to come back to see me prior to my surgery. So there she came, feeling relieved that she was able to see me. She didn't stay long. She gave me a kiss and went back out with Bill and Joanne. It seemed like forever that I was waiting to go back for my surgery. Of course, I couldn't see the time, but I knew it's been long. As I was waiting, Dr. Warren appeared and asked how I was holding up. I told her I was fine and that I was ready. We were waiting for Dr. D before we could get started. Do you know that she stayed there with me until it was almost time to take me into the surgical room? That gave me such a sense of relief that she would be "watching over me."

They started to wheel me away. Brenda said she would see me when it was finished and that I was in good hands. After that, I don't remember too much—either the drugs were starting to work or I just don't remember.

I don't really remember waking up, but I do remember wheeling down the hallway. I told my mom that I would be smiling coming out of surgery, and so when they told me that my family was there, I made sure I had a smile on my face and that I waved to them. I was finally in my room, and they asked me to scoot over to the other bed. I did it, but I certainly don't know how. Once they got me all settled in, my family came in. Bill, Brenda, Joanne, Mom, and Dad were all at the end of my bed. I remember them asking me questions and asking if they could take a peek. I, of course, said yes because I wanted to see it as well. To my surprise, there was not that much bandaging, and even though the breasts were gone, I still had a little mound where the expanders were placed. The drugs were still working well at that point. They could see that I was still pretty out of it so they did not stay long but made sure that I was okay before leaving. It was very hard for Bill to leave, but I tried to reassure him that I would be okay. He kissed me, and off he went.

The night seemed to go well, I was in a room with four beds, but only two were occupied. I was closest to the door, which was a good thing because it was closer to the bathroom. When I finally woke up and the meds had worn off, the nurse came to check on me. I told her that I had to use the bathroom, and she asked me if I thought that I could walk there. I was pretty nervous, but I knew that I was going to have to move at some point. I made it without too much discomfort and was glad that I took that first step. When I got back to the bed, I was given more pain medication. I was given "dinner," and afterwards, I watched some TV. I was in and out pretty much all night, and the discomfort was tolerable.

Saturday, September 15, 2007

Well, I made it through the night, and then came my breakfast. Oh yummy. I was able to call the kids and let them know I was okay; it was so good to hear their voices. I still think they are handling this very well. Bill said that he would be up after lunch to get me. After he had gotten off of the phone with me, he had sent out this email:

Hello, everyone, it's Bill, Sharon's husband. I just wanted to keep everyone informed of Sharon's prognosis.

She had her surgery yesterday, and everything went well. The doctors did find that her sentinel node contained cancer and another node was not normal. The final pathology report will be in at the doctor's office in seven to ten days. The treatment, if only the two nodes are affected, will be chemotherapy; and this can start in as soon as three weeks. Sharon is still Sharon, but on drugs. Her attitude is still very positive and she swears to have a promising future with all of this.

We are staying tonight at Brenda's so she can show me how to be a nurse and I can take care of her during the next few weeks. I don't know when she will be up to taking phone calls, but for now, she does not want to talk on the phone. I will be home if you would like to call, but she probably will not feel like talking. All we really need from everyone right now is your prayers. The next several months will be a rough road, but we will shift our lives into four-wheel drive and get over any more bumps that come our way.

Thanks for everyone who has called, sent gifts, and made prayers. We appreciate everyone's support. As information becomes available, you will be receiving updates.

Bill Hart, Jr.

As I was sitting there, my roommate had a check from her doctor, and she was going over some recovery instructions. She had not been able to get out of bed yet, and she was in a lot of pain. That was when I realized that she had the tram done. *Ouch!* I was so glad to be able to get up and use the bathroom, and somehow it made my pain/discomfort even less. Dr. Warren had come to check on me and was happy with what she saw. I thanked her for what she had done and looked forward to seeing her for my checkup. I never heard or saw Dr. D during the whole process; I guess she was there yesterday. Bill and Brenda arrived and informed me that the kids were with Joanne, and they were fine. As we are carefully getting dressed, I was thankful I remembered my button down shirt.

I am feeling pretty good. I am being cautious but at the same time courageous. The nurse went over all of the discharge papers, got my wheelchair, and told Bill he could go get the car. I got into the wheelchair and went for my chariot ride to the door. Bill was there, and he helped me into the car. I sat in the back of the van, and they had a pillow for me to put on my chest so that the seatbelt doesn't push into my chest. The ride home was fine, a little bumpy, but of course, you are more aware of bumps when you don't want to feel anything. Brenda took a picture on her phone and sent it to my mom and Joanne. Buddy has a baseball game today, and Joanne was taking him to that. We are trying to keep things as normal as possible for the kids. Joanne is going to need a spa day after all this is done. She has helped out with kids so much.

Bill dropped us off at Brenda's house, helped me get situated inside, and then went to fill my prescriptions. When I looked around, I noticed that Brenda has the house all cozy. Her couch was so comfortable, and she had the best pillows and blankets. And then there were some flowers for me. She has a Bassett Hound, Dudley, but she took him down to my mom's so that he wouldn't jump on me. He seems to think he is a lap dog.

Brenda was situating my supplies for emptying the drains and getting a spot for my meds and a piece of paper for documenting. I have to write down how much fluid we empty from my drains, and we are writing down when I take my meds. Bill returned with the happy pills and stayed for a while. He is handling this well, and I can tell he is so worried for me. My mom came up later that day and had bought me a beautiful pink pajama set. The top is button-down, of course. I got changed into them, and as I was doing that, I take a look at myself and think, *Not too bad-looking*. There were very few bandages and many tubes. I have three drains—two on my left side and one on my right side. Then I have a fanny pack around my waist with a very thin catheter that is inserted on each side of the chest. This is my On-Q ball which has Marcaine (an anesthetic) that sprays out on a constant basis to help reduce the pain. I am going to say that it is working nicely because the pain has not been that bad. I am also on Percocet, so that helps as well. It is not time to empty the drains yet, and I am sure glad that we are at Brenda's for this. It is a weird feeling to have a tube in you. You are afraid to move or touch it because you don't want it to fall out.

I have talked to the kids, and they seemed to be doing fine. They just wanted to know when I was coming home. They were spending the night with Joanne because Bill wanted to stay with me at Brenda's. I have not been the best company due to the Percocet that was making me pretty drowsy. It was around seven in the evening, and we decided that it was time to empty the drains. We got all ready by putting down a pad on my lap in case of spills. We lined up the three numbered bottles, got our paper out, and started to empty the drains. There is a ball at the end of the tube, which I have safety pinned to my "fanny pack" so they do not hang and pull so much. You have to open the top of the ball and just empty out the fluid. Before you close the top, you have to squeeze the ball and then close the top. This creates a suction so the fluid will drain. Once that is done, you see how much has drained, document it, and empty it in the toilet. Drain number one had fifty milliliters, drain number two had fifteen milliliters, and drain number three had forty milliliters. You want to see fluid like this because this is how it reduces the swelling. Every now and then, you have to "milk" the tubing to make sure there is no clogging going on. Now, that is gross. We all did well with our first of many sessions with this. We drained again at eleven in the evening and called it a night. I was on one couch, Bill was on the other one, and Brenda had gone up to her bed. She did offer me her bed, but due to the couch being so comfortable, I was content there.

I have had many people e-mailing me about the updates that I have been sending. There are some really inspiring messages, and I will be putting some of these in throughout the journal. But this one was written from my husband the day after my surgery, which I didn't read it until days later:

> *Punkin,*
>
> *I just wanted to send you an email to let you know that my love has grown tenfold for you over the last month. Your attitude, personality, and character are things I can not describe. I just want to also let you know that we are in this together, and I will be there every step of the way. It will be a long journey, but we will make it!*
>
> *Last night (Friday night) was one of the longest nights I have ever spent in my life. I thought the night would never end. Not having you next to me was something I never want to experience again. The boys were great company and helped me get through it.*
>
> *Seeing you in the hospital felt like I was the one having the surgery. Every muscle in my body hurt. I am accepting the fact, but don't be surprised if you see me at some point hit my bottom. I have a strange way of coping with things, but I will try my hardest to open up to you for support since we are in this together. I just don't want you to see me hurting because I do not want to get you down or your attitude*

to change. You need to stay positive and get through this stuff, and knowing you, it will happen.

    Anytime, day or night, I will be there for you.

I love you with all my heart.

Love,
Hubby

Sunday, September 16, 2007

I woke up about half past four in the morning. It was time to take my antibiotic and pain meds. Bill was right there with me, and we emptied the drains successfully. Back to la-la land I went. It takes the Percocet about twenty minutes before I can feel myself getting loopy, but I have been told not to be the superhero and try to hold off on them for the first couple of days. Being comfortable and relaxing is the main thing you want to do.

Later this morning, Bill decided that he better head home to spend some time with the kids and to get the house cleaned. I was supposed to go home with him but decided to stay at Brenda's for one more night. He is off tomorrow, so once he gets the kids off to school, he would come up and get me, bring me home, and get situated there before the kids get home from school.

Later on in the day, Brenda asked if I would like to wash up. So we headed to the bathroom and did a little sponge bath. She is such a good nurse. Since I was feeling good, she asked me if I wanted to get my hair washed. So we went to the sink and put a pillow over my chest, and I leaned over to get my hair washed. It was not painful, and we were doing great. Right before she got finished, I started feeling a little funny; but I thought I would be okay, and I didn't say anything. Then I told her that I feel like I need to sit down. We went to the bathroom. I sat down and I started feeling worse, I was getting hot and very nauseated. She told me to put my head between my legs as much as I could and put a cold cloth on my neck. After a few minutes I felt back to normal. I had some color back in me, and the nauseous feeling has gone away. We decided that I should hold off on blow drying my hair and go back to the couch and lie down for a while. Of course, she took a picture of me, and later on, we were laughing about it. That was not a good feeling, but it was nice to get cleaned up.

The rest of the day was pretty uneventful. That night, I did go upstairs to sleep in a real bed, and to my surprise, Brenda had an awesome arrangement of flowers up there as well. Her bedroom had an Oriental theme, and the flower arrangement had that same theme. She had my pillows situated, and there was this one pillow that was like the memory foam, but thicker, and it had been great for support. Maybe she would let me take it home tomorrow. Before we went to sleep, we emptied the drains, and drain number one had twenty milliliters, drain number two had ten milliliters, and drain number three had thirty milliliters. So things were slowing down some. Brenda and I talked for a little bit, and I realized how nice it is to be able to have some one-on-one time with her. We don't seem to do that like we should. I told her how much I have appreciated her being there for me. She has made these past couple of days very comfortable for me, so much that I almost didn't want to go home tomorrow. Family is a wonderful thing!

Monday, September 17, 2007

Brenda had to work today, so I headed downstairs and got comfortable on the couch. Prior to her leaving, she emptied the drains, got my meds, and got me some breakfast. During the time that we were checking the surgical site, I noticed a little blue bubble on my left "breast." It looked like it had fluid in it, and I showed it to Brenda. She was unsure of what it might be but told me not to pop it. We jokingly said that they must have given me a blue nipple as a surprise. We covered the site, and I got comfortable. I know that she would rather stay home with me, but she was coming down after work tonight. Prior to her leaving, she told me that I could borrow that pillow that I love so much.

Bill was coming to pick me up around ten in the morning, and I was sure I would be napping until he arrives. I have been noticing that when I take these little catnaps, I am really relaxed. I woke up, and my mouth was all open, and I have woken myself up by making these funky snoring noises! How embarrassing.

Bill came in and was very happy to see me and told me that I looked good. I got dressed and gathered my things, but I left the flowers with a little note in her bedroom, because they look so nice in her room. We got situated in the car and headed home.

When we got there, I found out that Bill had the couch all ready for me, but I decided to lie back in the bedroom for a little while. My dog, Darla, was very excited to see me; and she has not left my side. I got back into my pajamas and went to sleep. Prior to the kids getting home, I moved out on the couch. Bill had already informed them that when they see me, they have to be very careful. Their hugs are going to have to be a squeeze on the hand or arm.

They finally got home, and the smiles on their face are priceless. They gave me hugs and wanted to see where I got cut. They were amazed with all of the tubes that were on me. I kind of felt like a bionic woman or a cow with utters! My niece Jessica got home shortly after the boys, and she has been anxious to take care of me. She was not as interested to see the tubes right then, but she would come around. I have felt very strongly about being very open with the kids. I do not want to hide anything from them, and I want them to feel comfortable with asking questions. I feel that if you hide things from them, they will think things are worse than they really are or that they can't talk to you about it.

Later on that night, Bill took Buddy to Cub Scouts, and my mom, Joanne, and Brenda stayed with me. Joanne and Mom told me how funny it was when they came in the house yesterday. Bill had been telling us how much he had cleaned the house, and when they came over, they were shocked to see what was not done. Don't get me wrong; he tried really hard and did a lot, but it is amazing what clean means to a man versus a woman. You gotta love 'em. Brenda's friend, little Brenda, had made an apple pie for us to enjoy, so we tried a piece; but we needed some ice cream to go with it. Bill came home and everyone left shortly after that. Brenda told me that she could stop by on Wednesday to check on me and help me with a shower. Bill got the kids ready for bed and got me situated in our bed. He has not been sleeping with me because he is nervous that he is going to roll over and try to hug me; and he doesn't want to hurt me. I pretty much don't move during the night due to the drains, but again, he was being so thoughtful. He kissed me goodnight and told me to wake him if I need anything. I watched a little TV, and then for some reason, I had an emotional moment. I was just thinking of how helpless I was feeling right then, and I couldn't do anything about it. It is very hard to go from doing so much to not being able to do or help with anything. I got myself together and went on to watch some TV.

Tuesday, September 18, 2007

It was a good night. The kids give me their "hugs" before going to school, and I told them to have a great day. Since Zachary is in preschool, Bill has to take him, which means he has to leave me by myself. I am okay with this, but he does not like it. I reassured him that I was going to be okay and he would be back shortly. He gave me a big "hug" and didn't want to let go. I did go out on the couch while he was gone, and I had noticed that my On-Q ball was deflated. So I checked the instructions, and I remembered Dr. Warren saying that when it is out, I just have to pull the catheters out. They are long but so small that I probably won't need a Band-aid. When Bill came home, he informed me that everyone was asking about me and told me that they were thinking of me. I informed him that we had to do some surgery. It was time to remove two of the "tubes." We were feeling a little nervous but knew that we could do it. I had to help him get the tape off since he has short fingernails, and then he started to pull out the first catheter. It was pretty long and so skinny that I didn't even feel it coming out. Even though I didn't really need a Band-aid, we put one on anyway. It felt good to have a couple of tubes gone. The fanny pack could come off, but I decided to leave it on because I have my drains pinned to that. This way, when I go to the bathroom, I wouldn't have to unpin them from my pants everytime. My blue "nipple" was still there and was a little bigger. I have an appointment with Dr. Warren on Thursday, and I will just get it checked then. I am being careful not to pop it.

The day went by, and not too much was happening. I was feeling good and getting hooked on the cooking channel. How I would love to have a kitchen like that and be able to cook some of those things. It has worked out great this week because Bill is on his seven-day break. I have tried to get him to go and do what he has to do, but it is so hard for him to leave me. I am still trying to get him to open up to me, but it is hard for him. Everytime he leaves, he puts his head face down on my arm and stays there for about five minutes. I give him his time and continue to reassure him that it will be okay.

Another friend stopped by and dropped off a dinner for us. It is a wonderful thing to have friends step up to the plate in a time of need. We enjoyed the dinner and had some family time together. The drains continued to slow down, and the kids were helping me with emptying and measuring them. I don't have to empty them as often as I had to. The kids got ready for bed, and they gave me their goodnight "hugs". Bill tucked me in and went to the couch. I had another breakdown tonight, but this time, it was because I couldn't hug the boys and Bill like I wanted to. I never realized how much a hug can do for one person.

Wednesday, September 19, 2007

My friend Debbie visited me and brought me dinner. It was nice to sit and talk with her, and she told me that I looked great. During her stay, I received some flower deliveries. My house smelled so nice. I have taken pictures of all the flowers that have come in; they were all so beautiful. I am still taking the Percocet, but I am waiting a little longer in between doses. I am happy to say that I have not had a lot of pain. My right arm has more mobility and less numbness. The left arm gets more stabbing pains in the armpit, and it is really numb. So the shaving will have to be put on hold for a little while (imagine that site), and it is hard putting on deodorant without looking in the mirror. So if you come around me on a hot day, watch out!

Brenda came over tonight to help me get a shower and to check on things. You wouldn't think it is hard, but these dag on drains are a pain in the you-know-what. I am feeling refreshed and am looking forward to my appointment with Dr. Warren tomorrow. I might be getting the drains out.

I didn't have a breakdown tonight. I think I felt so refreshed and relaxed and actually felt like I accomplished something that I was able to fall right asleep.

Thursday, September 20, 2007

I had my appointment to get my drains out today at 2:00 p.m. Bill was going to get some grass cut first, and then he would be back in time for the appointment. Chrissy stopped by and dropped off dinner and a cake. She stayed with me for a while, which made Bill a little more comfortable. I asked her how she has been feeling and if the pregnancy has settled in yet. She was feeling like a pregnant woman but was accepting it better. I showed her my surgical site, and she was amazed at how small the incision was and how good it looked. As you can see, I have no problem asking my friends if they want to see the site. I figured that if I was in their shoes, I would want to see it too but would not know if it was okay to ask. I want people to be aware of what happens and what to expect or know if, heaven forbid, they would have to go through this.

We were headed to Dr. Warren's, and it felt good to get out. I was not able to move the left arm so much, and I was feeling tight, but my drains were coming out today. Hooray! I was excited but nervous because I could remember when I had my drain pulled out of my knee back in 1988. It was gross. It is a feeling that you can't explain. It doesn't hurt; it is just nasty. As

I was sitting in the waiting room, I was thinking to myself, wondering how many people think I have just gotten a boob job and if they could see that I was not that comfortable. Little do they know that I had a boob job all right. During this process, I could see that I was going to learn a lot about myself. Those people were probably not even thinking any of that. That is what I would be thinking if I was sitting there, and it goes to show that you can't pass judgment on anyone because you don't really know the whole story.

Anyway, I got called back, and Dr. Warren examined me. She removed the surgi-strips that were on the site, and it looked amazing, considering what I have just had done. She saw my blue "nipple" and saw that there was fluid in it. When she removed some of the tape, she released the fluid from the "nipple" and said that she did not want infection to start by keeping it there. She informed me that it was not fungus like I was thinking it was; it was from the dye that they used to locate the nodes during surgery. The skin sometimes does not react nicely with the dye, so I had some blistering going on there. I just needed to use some antibiotic ointment and let the body heal itself. Then it was time for the drains to come out. She checked to see what the amounts were, and since yesterday at half past midnight to eight thirty in the morning today, drain number one had fifteen milliliters, drain number two had hardly any, and drain number three had twenty milliliter. She was happy with the slowing down and was ready to take them out. I informed her that I was nervous and might have to lie down. She laid me back anyway, and Bill couldn't wait to see them removed. He even asked if he could take one out! She of course said no but that he could come up and watch her remove them. The drains were kept in by some sutures, so she cut them and then started pulling it out. Yuck, the drain was pretty far in me and felt like it was wrapped around the expander. Like I said, it does not hurt, but you can feel the tube moving inside of you, and that is just gross. After seeing how far the drain was in me, I don't see why I was so worried of it coming out. Bill was amazed because he could see it moving in my skin as it was coming out. I told him that he was not helping me by being so verbal. She removed the next one from my left side, but that one was not in as much. It was where my lymph nodes were removed under my arm. I felt a little warm, and she went to the right side to remove the last one. This one was in pretty far as well. When she was finished, she sat me up, but I told her that I was feeling pretty warm and felt the need to lie back down. She got me a glass of water and let me get myself together. She told me that she would see me back in a week and that we may start filling the expanders. She gave me a prescription for the ointment to put on the blisters, and she would check that area as well. When I left, I was feeling much better, and again, I was so thankful to have such a great surgeon to be there for me.

I called and filled everyone in on what happened and went home to get some more rest. When I got home, there were more flowers that have been delivered, and the mailbox was full of cards. So I got into some comfortable clothes and surrounded myself with my flowers and read all the nice cards and things that friends and family had sent me.

The next couple of days went by, and I was trying to do a little more. I can't tell you how nice it is not to have the "utters" hanging. I feel like a new person. It was the weekend, and I was going with Joanne to my parents' house while she cuts my dad's hair. I feel the need to get out of the house for a little bit. My dad hasn't seen me in a couple of days, and you could tell that he was concerned about me but was glad to see me out.

We went back to Joanne's, and there came my friend Michelle dropping off a basket full of dinner and goodies to make ice cream sundaes. My sister was excited because she wouldn't have to fix dinner, and we jokingly said that we were going to start asking for double dinners because we were always together.

On Saturday, I went to Buddy's game, and everyone was surprised to see me. I figured that I would go since it was not anything strenuous, and the weather was nice. I thought Buddy and Zachary were glad to see me up and doing things as well. Later that night, Joanne hung out with me and the kids while Bill went down to Kelly's, a little bar in Port Penn. I felt that he needed a night out with the guys, and I think that he enjoyed himself.

Monday, September 24, 2007

I had my appointment with Dr. D for my results from the pathology report. My mom was off work so she was going to go with us. We got to the Breast Center for my appointment at 1:15 p.m. Once we checked in, we went and sat down and patiently waited, but after about forty minutes, we started to get anxious and wanted to see what the holdup was all about. When we asked how much longer it was going to be, they informed us that Dr. D was not even in that office today. They called her other office in Wilmington, and they informed us that our appointment was there at 1:15 p.m. I showed them the paper that the office sent me that said the Breast Center. They apologized and told us that we can set up another appointment, but we refused and told them that I needed to be seen today. My mom decided to go home due to the time, and Bill and I headed into Wilmington. We were not too happy at that point. I do understand that mistakes happen, but when we checked in, wouldn't you think that someone would have noticed that I wasn't on the book or that when I said that I was here for Dr. D, they would have said then that she wasn't there. Anyway, we finally got to the other office, and it was after two in the afternoon. We got taken back, and when she came in, she had an intern with her and asked if we minded that she was there during our visit. I told her that I didn't mind at all. She went into a very scientific and detailed report, but this is what we got out of it: They found that three out of the sixteen lymph nodes were positive with cancer. I thought they were going to say two, so I wasn't too far off. The surgery site looked good, the tumor size was pretty large, but the cancerous area measured three and a half centimeters in the breast. The border margins were not invasive; that was only in my breast. I would need to have chemo and radiation. I believe the radiation is more of preventive, but I would be seeing the radiation oncologist this Friday. I am going to need some physical therapy on the left arm due to scar tissue and tightness. She suggested that I have a chemo port placed due to the size of my veins. They already have trouble finding my veins, so having this port placed would make it easier when I get my chemo because they have to inject it through a vein. After giving all of the information, she asked if we had any questions. I informed her that I didn't have any questions but did have some concerns. I wanted to let her know about what had happened in today's visit and that I do understand mistakes, but the front-desk officer should be a little more careful for such an important appointment. I then went into how I was disappointed when I found out afterward that she never went out to my family after the surgery was over to let them know how everything went. They never heard anything until Dr. Warren had gone out to speak with them. She told me that since my sister was checking in on things, she assumed that she was letting everyone know. I told her that even though she was a nurse and she was checking in on me from her workplace, it was not her responsibility to come over and tell my family. I told her that I feel that she is a good surgeon (from what I can tell since I was asleep the whole time), but her communication needed some help. Also, being in the dental field, I know that if you are not informed at the front desk about what goes on, you may never know, and that hurts your business. I felt like what I gave her was constructive criticism, but she told me that no matter what she did, she did not feel as though she could do right for me. She did not thank me for letting her know what was going on with the lack of communication with her staff. When she was leaving the room, she told me that she would be more than happy to give me other names of people who could help me out. She started shaking her head in disgust and walked out. So, needless to say, when I left there, I felt she was done with me, and I was done with her. Maybe you could say that that was the day that I fired my general surgeon. I was very proud of Bill for keeping his cool during this whole visit, but I think we were both surprised with her reaction.

It was an emotional day for both of us—hearing about the lymph node involvement and dismissing your surgeon—but otherwise here are how things are going: *As far as the emotional side, I am still me and very positive with everything that is going on. I continue to counsel my family and help them through this. The hardest thing is not being able to play and love the kids like I want to, but I keep telling myself that it is only temporary. My hubby is getting better each day, very emotional in the beginning, and he is learning to share this with me as I have reassured him that it is not going to bring me down. My mom is great with her meds, and Joanne is getting stronger as it goes on. My dad—he is dad and doesn't say too much. Brenda, she is my right arm with all the medical information and support. The boys and my nieces are my sunshine. They ask me every day if I am getting better, and they are handling it well. I can't say enough how much I LOVE my family and how important it is to have a relationship with them. So my advice to you all is that if you have any grudges or differences with any of your family, make peace, move on, and love them. You never know what can happen and when you will need them.*

I would like to thank everyone for your thoughts, prayers, cards, flowers, fruits, and dinners! They have helped in more ways than you can imagine. It amazes me what friends you have in time of need, so again, I want to thank you!

Someone has told me that having cancer is like having a full-time job. I think I would have to agree, but there is one difference—you don't get paid for all of your hard work. You do however get paid with support and friendship, which I am getting overtime!

Hello Again.

Wednesday, September 26, 2007

I had a consultation today with another general surgeon. Even though there was no real need for one at this point, I would like to have one who knows my situation from the beginning. My appointment was at 1:00 p.m., and my dad was taking me since I was not able to drive due to limited movement. When I walked into the office, we definitely noticed how outdated the office was, but I was not judging her yet. When I was called back, the rooms were quite outdated as well. I got changed and waited for her to come in, and when she did, I think *don't judge a book by its cover* and how that is true. She was very interested in what was going on with me and was concerned with the "scab" that I have on my left breast. She did a thorough exam and asked if I would get dressed and meet her in her office. When I went to her office, she had all of my records and thoroughly went over what had been done so far. She did agree with the treatment that was done, and everything looked good. She did recommend that I get a second opinion from a medical oncologist. Not that there was a chance that I wouldn't need chemo but that I was going to have a long-term relationship with that person, and I should make sure that we "click." It wouldn't be too good if I fired my oncologist in the middle of treatment. I sound like I am such a hard person to get along with, not! She was going to see me back in about a month just to check on how things are going and if I have any questions or concerns. I was very pleased with her chairside manners and felt that she is there for her patients.

My dad took me home, and I rested for the remainder of the day. I continued to feel well, not a lot of pain, just tightness. I am hardly taking any Percocet, and as I stated, the blue area is no longer blue; it has now turned into a scab. I filled everyone in on the visit and waited for the next ones to come.

Thursday, September 27, 2007

I had an appointment with Dr. Warren, whom I always look forward to seeing due to her calm nature. We did not fill the water balloons this time. She said that I still feel a little tight, and we were in no hurry to complete this so we would wait until next week. A little bit of swelling on the right side, but not enough to drain. Thank goodness! I did express some tightness and lack of mobility, and she gave me an Rx for therapy with Specialty Rehabilitation on Main Street, Newark. Dr. Warren would see me next week.

Friday, September 28, 2007

Today, I met with Dr. Jon Strasser, the radiation oncologist. He seemed very nice and knowledgeable. He did recommend that I get radiation, more of a preventive measure. The protocol is that if there are four positive lymph nodes and the tumor size is five centimeters, then definitely there is a need for radiation, but he said that I was in the grey area. Due to my age and one of the nodes being irregularly shaped—meaning that some of the cancer cells broke outside of the node (but is not in my body)—he would recommend twenty-eight days of radiation, not including weekends. (Wasn't that nice of him?) This would not happen until after chemo is done, so I would not see him for a little while.

On this same day, I met with Dr. W, a medical oncologist. He suggested that I do all three meds at the same time (can't remember the names) during a morning session (four hours) and then come back the next day for a booster shot to raise my white-blood-cell count and then not return for three weeks. We would do this six times, which would be a total of eighteen weeks, if you are not too good in math. He gave me an Rx for a hair prosthesis! What color should I get? This is my time to experiment. He doesn't think that my side effects will be too bad because I am young and strong. He did recommend that I get a chemo port placed. He also recommended Dr. S. I also need a chest X-ray, blood test, and some tests to check my heart. Prior to my leaving, they tried to schedule all of this, but I did not make any of the appointments because I have a second-opinion appointment scheduled with Dr. Biggs on Thursday, which of course I will fill you in on.

Saturday, September 29, 2007

I had my consultation today at Specialty Rehabilitation. The office is on the small side but very nicely decorated. It almost looks like a spa but with exercise equipment. I filled out my paperwork and waited to be called back. When I got back to the room, I noticed that it has a massage table in the middle. They asked that I put on a gown. The nice thing about these gowns is that they are not the normal hospital gown material; they are regular patterns. I would have to let her know how nice that was. It is just the little things that you don't think make a difference, but they do. Lisa, the owner, came in and introduced herself and gathered some information about my past. She informed me that ninety-five percent of their patients are cancer patients, hence the name Specialty Rehab, and that they would take good care of me. She was very informative. Every time I meet someone, I learn more and more. My mom was with me, and of course, she heard that I am not supposed to lift anything heavier than five pounds, so I can't even break it because she (mom) has emphasized to my family about that little comment. Did you know that a gallon of milk weighs eight pounds? I will continue to see her for the next four weeks, longer if needed. During the consultation, she looked at the surgical site and was surprised with the size of my breasts already without any fills. I told her that I was a DD and had a lot of skin prior to surgery! She looked surprised, and then I told her the truth, and she found that funny. But for those of you who have not seen me, I am about an A and a half. She finished with the appointment by going over some stretches to do, and she will see me back early next week. My mom and I really like her and feel that it is a place for me. It seems that they are definitely there for the patients.

Monday, October 1, 2007

Bill was on day work, and I got the boys off to school. I got my genetic testing results today at nine in the morning. I was taking a tape recorder with me since Bill was unable to go, and I may not remember all of the specifics. Marcie called me, and we went into the same room where she spoke about genetic testing with me before. I asked if she minds that I record everything, and she said it was fine. I saw the envelope in front of her, and I felt like it is the Grammy's. Am I going to be the winner? Guess what? We have some great news! I won the Grammy today. I do not have the BRCA I or BRCA II gene. YEAH! This is very good news for me and my family because it does not automatically put them at a higher risk for getting breast cancer.

The meeting was short because of this, and there was no real need to leave the tape recorder running. I thanked her for the good news and went out to tell my dad, who was my chauffeur today. Even though my dad does not show a lot of emotions, I know that he was happy to hear this news especially for my mom because she was very nervous about what could be in store for her. Even though I tried to reassure her that even if it was positive it would be okay, Mom is still Mom and worries herself.

On to our next appointment, which is my second visit with the therapist, and oh did she stretch me! The numbness was what was uncomfortable. She gave me more stretches and massaged me some. She was running late, but good old dad sat waiting patiently. The funny thing was when I was at the desk to make another appointment, they apologized for the wait and hoped that my husband didn't mind! I started to laugh and corrected them by saying that he was my dad.

When we finished, we went to lunch at Bennigans, went to the K-mart, Dollar Store, and then called it a day. We laughed, thinking how many other people thought we were husband and wife. It was nice going shopping and spending a little money since the only money that has been spent was for the doctors. The even better thing was that my dad and I are getting to spend more time together! I know I have said it before, but family is a great thing.

Here I am again.

Wednesday, October 3, 2007

I had another physical therapy appointment, and again I learned more stretches, and it went well. My dad was my chauffeur again, but I can see that we are not going to be allowed to be out together very often. We were gone all day. We went to Milburn Orchards and got some fruit and other items, to Kohls (short period, if that is possible), to the bank, to Happy Harry's, and then came home. My mom was giving us a hard time (in a joking way) because she couldn't get in touch with us. We may be dangerous together, but it is fun.

Later that night, my sisters and I went to a breast cancer survivor reception/seminar at the Waterfall on Philadelphia Pike. It was very nice; we of course had some excitement while we were there. An older man (a breast cancer survivor; yes, it can happen to men) was sitting next to me during the refreshments. He was in a dead stare at Joanne, and the next thing I know, he started to fall over towards me! I held him up even though I am not supposed to be lifting weights heavier than five pounds and called for Brenda who was standing behind me. He was very sweaty and pale. They took off his jacket and put a cold rag on him, and he started to regain consciousness! They called an ambulance, but, of course, he did not want to go to. He blamed the incident on his alcohol beverage.

We went into the seminar room, where the guest speaker was Wendi Fox-Pedicone, author of "Hangin' Out With Lab Coats." She is such an inspirational person and speaker. She is a breast cancer survivor but recently had a relapse and is now considered terminal. (Don't be nervous, her cancer was more advanced than mine is, not to say that I can't relapse, but all cases are different.) The cancer has gone to her liver and lungs. If you look at her, you would never know that she is terminal. She looks thin and her hair, yes, she has hair, is thin. But she has such confidence and inspiration. I hoped to meet her this evening.

During the seminar, two rows in front of us, a lady took her jacket off; and next thing we know, her head was tilted back, and she sounded like she was snoring. NOT! She has passed out! They paused the seminar, put her on the ground, and she became conscious. The ambulance came and took her to the hospital. My sisters and I looked at each other and asked, "Is it us?"

I asked a friend next to me if it was us, and she laughed and said, "No, but I will say that in the years that I have come here, this has never happened!" Go figure.

Anyway, we had a great evening, and if you want another good book to read, you should try it. I did get to meet Wendi at the end of the evening, and she was happy to meet me and told me to e-mail her at anytime. It was very nice being together with my sisters; we seem to always cause a ruckus. By the end of the night, I was very tired and ready for bed. I was feeling pretty bruised and felt as though I needed to take a Percocet. Off to la-la land I went.

Thursday, October 4, 2007

I started my day with an appointment with Dr. Warren, my sister Joanne, and niece Jaylyn went with me. Joanne was very curious, and she came back with me. I had the steri-strips removed. I know it should have hurt, but because I was still numb, I didn't feel a thing. Dr. Warren continued to be happy with the healing. She got the syringe ready for my first fill of the water balloons. She found the entry site by a magnet, marked it with a pen, and gave a little anesthesia. It hurts a little. She then injected the needle, which I felt. She said it was going through the muscle, and that is what I was feeling. Did you get a little twinge reading that statement? I want you to feel as though you are getting it done. HA-HA! Anyway, I could feel it getting tighter. She pulled out the syringe and went to the other side. We were now thirty CC's larger. What does that make me? An "A and three quarters"? She said I would be tight again just as I was getting used to it! Oh well! Joanne and Jaylyn did very well with the whole process. Even though my niece is only three years old, I have been very open to her about what is going on. She doesn't really understand, but she knows that Aunt Sharon has a boo-boo on her boobie and that I am getting it all better. The last thing that I would want is for her or anyone to be afraid if it was to happen to them.

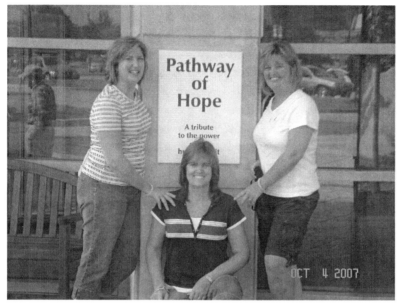

Brenda, Myself and Joanne in front of the Helen Graham Center

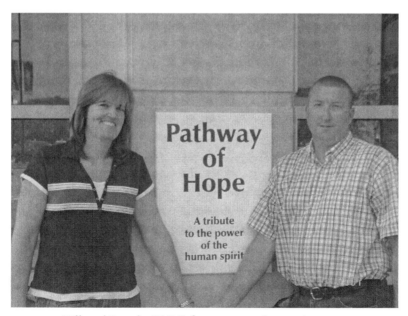

Bill and I at the HGC for my consult appointment

Later today, I had my appointment for my second opinion with Dr. Biggs, a medical oncologist. Bill and both my sisters came with me to this one. He was very nice; he examined me, asked me to get dressed and asked me to meet him in his office. That won me over right there. Any doctor who will take the time to talk to you in his office versus the operatory is a good doctor in my opinion! We all went into his office, and I turned my tape recorder on. I need help remembering now with all of this information I have been getting. He explained everything very thoroughly and felt that the treatment option to go with is the sixteen-week cycle, getting treatments every two weeks. The first four weeks would be "Adriamycin and Cytoxin," and the following four weeks would be "Taxol."

He chose this treatment versus the three-week one because studies show that young women with a high-grade tumor have done better. He explained that I would come in on a Wednesday, get blood work, see him, and then come back on a Thursday for the actual chemo. (The first four weeks take about one and a half hours, and the second four weeks take about four to five hours). On a Friday, I would go in for a white blood cell booster shot. I should lose my hair on my head approximately three weeks after the first dose of chemo, later for the rest of my hair. Oh boy, no more shaving! He wanted me to get the port done, have a MUGA scan to check the heart, have a "chemo talk" with the nurse about side effects, etc., and start treatment on Wednesday, October seventeenth! He gave me my prescriptions for nausea and my cranial prosthetic (wig) and wanted me to get my first blood work so that on Wednesday, we can start the chemo. The other treatments will be like I explained earlier, but this time, since it is my first treatment, they can check my blood work now. The reason for the blood work is to check your counts and make sure it is okay to get the chemo. But since I am just starting, my counts are good to go. The doctor also discussed with me about being in a blind study using an herb or vitamin, can't remember, that may reduce the amount of side effects during treatment. You need to do a good amount of documentation during the process, and I may not even be the one who takes it. That is how a blind study works—the one giving the meds and the one taking the meds don't know if it is the real "stuff." I don't think I am interested; I have enough things to remember, and if I have to write a lot of stuff down, I probably wouldn't do it. Anyway, I went and met Dr. Biggs's receptionist, and she got all of my appointments set up. Obviously, I am comfortable with Dr. Biggs, and I like his bedside manners, so he is officially my medical oncologist. As I have learned a little too late, don't be afraid to get a second opinion.

I went to get the blood test, and we headed home. Another busy day! When we got home, there was a phone call from Dr. Biggs stating for me to call his office tomorrow because he forgot to mention something to me. Oh great! I have to wait all night for this.

I continued to feel bruised today, and it was hard to laugh. I am doing pretty well, but I am being hard on myself and would like to be one hundred percent fine. I know that is not possible right now. The therapy is helping and the therapist is great! I continue to get my rest but not so much that I am getting lazy even though that would be easy to do. We continue to have some emotional roller coasters, but we all get through them together. It is an eye-opening experience, but my family and friends continue to be there for me. My boys are continuing to handle this pretty well. They still know that they have to be careful with the hugs and that I am getting ready for medicine that is going to make me pretty sick and that my hair is going to fall out. Which they think is pretty funny. Being open about cancer and treatments is the biggest key in getting through this tough time. If you hold things in, they will build up on you and explode, not the healthiest thing to happen. You have other "explosives" in your body, you don't need to add to them.

Friday, October 5, 2007

It was a rough night's sleep just wondering what Dr. Biggs forgot to tell me, but I called him first thing in the morning. Dr. Biggs got on the phone and just wanted me to be aware that during chemo, some women have their menstrual cycle and don't miss a beat or they may stop for a period of time. It could be up to two years. Other women go into early menopause, which means that if I am planning on having any more children, I can freeze my eggs. Oh no, another decision! I am happy with my two boys, and if I can't have any more, I will be okay with that. Not having my menstrual period is like not having to buy diapers anymore. I know some of you may be jealous—new set of breasts, no more shaving (for a time period), and possibly no more menstrual period! Although I wouldn't suggest this route for anyone!

Later today, the whirlwind began! Dr. Biggs called me again and informed me that my liver enzymes came back abnormal and that he wanted me to get a CAT scan to check my liver! He stated that it could be a couple of things—alcohol intake (NOT), aspirin (possibly from Percocet, but he doesn't feel like I have taken enough), some other reasons, but worst-case scenario is that the breast cancer has moved to my liver! WHAT, I couldn't be hearing this right. He wanted me to get the test today so that he could get the results before he leaves next week (vacation). It was a quarter past ten in the morning, and I needed to be there by 11:15 a.m. to drink this stuff for the CAT scan scheduled at 1:15 p.m. Bill was in Upper Derby doing a coverup for a fire department that was going to a fireman's funeral. Yesterday, he asked if he could go and since I had no doctors' appointment and my past couple of days were busy, this would give me and him a time to relax—not. I got in touch with my "sister" (long-time family friend) Stacey, and she was available to take me. I was pacing back and forth, praying to God that it was wrong! I informed Bill to stay at the coverup because there was nothing that he could do if he comes home. Stacey would be with me, and we wouldn't get the results until later tonight. He must have called twenty times during the day to check on me. We finally got there. I got my "tasty smoothie", and we sat outside by the fountain and talked. The smoothie was not too tasty; and lo and behold, during that time, I had to go to the bathroom. I am noticing a pattern here—when my nerves kick in, something needs to come out.

It was finally time for the CAT scan. I was a little nervous because I kept remembering the MRI. I got my gown on, and the nurse asked for me to sit on the chair. She needs to put an IV in for the dye. I informed her that I am a hard stick, but she did real well. I lay in the machine. The opening was much bigger, and the tube was shorter than the MRI. She informed me that when the dye is put through, I would get a warm sensation, and it may feel like I have to pee, but I wouldn't. I went back and forth through the tube. She wanted my arms to be above my head, but I couldn't do it due to limited mobility so I had to hold them up and rest my hands on my head. She asked me, through a microphone, to hold my breath, which I didn't think I would be able to do because of the nerves, but I did survive. There was a little break in between as they were waiting for the dye to get to my bladder. It finally did, and I went through it one more time, and I was complete. I went and got dressed, and Stacey and I went up to Biggs's office, wondering if I should wait for the results. But she said he would look at them after hours, and that would be after 4:40 p.m. We sat in the car for a little while and waited for a phone call, and then we decided it would be better to head home.

We ordered Chinese, like we think that we were going to be able to eat! We picked up her son and the food, headed to my house, and waited patiently. We were sitting down, trying to eat, and the phone rang. I saw that it was Dr. Biggs. I went into the bedroom, and he informed me that there is no sign of metastasis! Everyone took a deep breath; we have more good news. He then said that it could have been a faulty test or that I could have contracted hepatitis. I have had the series of shots and the booster, but that is not a guarantee, so he wanted me to get a retest on Monday. My family and friends all had a sigh of relief, and I will tell you, today was a very long day, but I am glad about the results.

Later that night, I was mentally drained, and all I could do was lie in my bed. My hubby and Joanne took the kids to "Frightland" and allowed me to be alone. It did help, but I do not suggest doing that for long periods of time as depression will set in quickly. I got my emotions together and caught up on some shuteye before they returned. The kids brought me a stuffed animal that they had won, and off to bed I was.

Well, as usual, it is never a dull moment in the life of the Harts at this particular time. I have given you more information for you to think about. I do feel as though you all are going through this journey with me. We are all hanging in there, and we will get through this trying time. Keep up the positive thoughts and prayers. Go enjoy your family and loved ones, and don't worry yourself about ever getting this dreaded disease. If it comes, you worry about it then.

Monday, October 8, 2007

I had a very good weekend, and now it is back to the sticks and pricks. I had to go to the HGC to get a retest for my liver. Tawanna was my nurse, and when she stuck me, I didn't feel a thing. LOVE HER! This was to check my hepatitis status.

IT'S ME AGAIN.

Tuesday, October 9, 2007

It was another therapy session, and it was going nicely. She did forewarn me that I would go two steps forward and one step back and not to get discouraged! Bill went on a field trip with Buddy at school and then took me to therapy. I was getting my port placed tomorrow so nothing to eat or drink after midnight.

Wednesday, October 10, 2007

Since we had to be at Christiana Hospital by 7:30 a.m., we had our neighbor put Buddy on the bus, we took Zachary to school, and we headed to the Heart and Vascular center. We didn't know where we were going or who we were seeing. I did know one thing—if I ever need to be regulated, I just need to go to a doctor's appointment. I can tell you where every bathroom is. Nerves, I tell you! We signed in, and I was taken back. The lady told Bill she would be out to get him as soon as I was prepped. Almost an hour later, which didn't seem like that to me, they finally brought Bill back. He was not too happy since it took so long. I was doing my regular talking and questioning since I was going into this blind. The doctor's nurse practitioner came in and explained the whole process of the port placement. While she was doing this, the nurse was trying to get the IV in me without hurting me too much. She found a spot on the side of my hand, and the vein was rolling. Doesn't that sound like fun? Anyway, the question came up about where the port should be placed—chest or arm. Sue said she would ask the doctor and would be right back. She returned with the answer being in my arm due to the expanders that are already present. I was ready to go, and they wheeled me away. Bill was trying to find a way for him to come into the operating room because he wanted to see what they do, but it didn't work. I went in, and I found it really weird that I could see everything that was going on. They were setting up the room and talking to me, and I was having fun with them as usual. Apologizing for my hairy and stinky underarms! Dr. K came in, introduced himself, and explained the procedure and what would be done. He stepped out, and they gave me a light anesthesia. I started to feel a little loopy, and then it went away. I thought to myself, *I hope that they do not start because I felt as if I was completely coherent.* I don't even remember the doctor coming back in, so the anesthesia must have been working. They gave me a little more, and I could feel some pressure and pushing. They were checking with me, asking me if I was okay and telling me that they were almost done. They also told me that they did not have to give me as much anesthesia due to my CALMNESS. I could have fallen asleep during the procedure, but I was too nosey and wanted to hear what they were doing and saying. As I left the operating room, I felt fine. Bill came in and did not expect me to be so alert. The nurses got me adjusted and gave me "breakfast," which was hard pancakes and nasty eggs. As she explained, they had to microwave them so I had to eat them fast. About five minutes later, she said that lunch has been delivered, and she gave me that tray as well. It was an open-faced hot turkey sandwich, green beans, and a salad with apple juice. Much better! I had to stay in the recovery room for forty-five minutes. I went for a little walk to check my steadiness, and then I could leave. All was well, and of course, when I went to put my button-up blouse on, the button fell off right at the breast area! The nurse and I paper-clipped it, and I was on my way. Since I was feeling pretty good, and there was a breast cancer awareness event going on at the medical arts pavilion, we went over and checked it out. To my surprise, Wendi from the book was doing signings. I went up to her, and she remembered me from the other night. She signed my book and told me to keep in touch. She is such an inspiration! After that, we headed out, and I ran into the nurse who did my ultrasound and mammogram. I knew that I knew her from somewhere, but that day was a little fuzzy. We headed home, and I rested for the remainder of the day.

October 11, 2007

Today was one of those busy doctor days. I needed to be at the Medical Arts Pavilion, so I thought, by 10:00 a.m., for my MUGA scan. When we checked in, we sat there for a while, and then the receptionist informed us that we should be at the Christiana Hospital. We headed over there, not too happy about this, of course, since our paper did say Medical Arts Pavilion. I felt like I was having a déjàvu! Anyway, we went over to check in, explained why we were late, and went and sat down. The receptionists called my name to come back, and I saw the dreaded blood-drawing chair! I asked her if I had to get a stick, and she informed me yes and for two times. I started to feel nervous and told her that I was a hard stick. I informed her of my port that was placed yesterday, and she let me know that they don't like to use them due to the possibility of the fluid that they inject sticking to the tubing of the port. Fine by me because I don't think I was telling her that to make her try and stick me there. I just wanted her to know that I had the port placed yesterday. She started looking for a vein, and she was having problems. She went and got another nurse, and she tried in the crease of my arm. She thought she got it, but when she administered the saline, it was burning, which means that it was not in the vein. So she pulled it out. She asked me if I have eaten or drank anything today, and I informed her that I had a pop tart and some water. She got a warm compress and checked my hand. She stuck me in the hand, and at that point, I was breaking down. I was trying to hold back, but it was not working. Bill couldn't even look at me, and when I thought she had it, she pulled out and says she couldn't get it. Now, Bill has had enough and asked if we could just reschedule. My veins have been poked at so much in the past couple of days that we needed a break! The nurse noted that we could reschedule for Monday. The nurses were apologetic, but I informed them it was not their fault. They tried. As we went to reschedule, one of the receptionists asked me if I was okay; and I broke down again, stating that it was my nerves and that Bill was going to have to schedule the appointment for me. I walked out, and the ladies stated that they felt like giving me a hug. Bill informed them that that probably wasn't a good idea right then. He later told me that he was about to break down and felt horrible that he didn't run right after me, but he knew that I needed my space. I calmed down and told him that it was just overwhelming! You don't get to recover from one surgery/procedure before they set you up for another one!

After that, we headed over to the Helen Graham Center for the "chemo talk." The talk was a lot of information that I do not want to bore you or confuse you with. Basically, it was about preventive treatment, what not to eat, what meds to take, etc. It was a very long discussion. The nurse then looked at the port because I was concerned with the redness. She had another nurse look at it. She felt that there may be some infection, and that I should have it checked just to be safe. So, we headed back over to the vascular center, and the nurse practitioner looked at it. She said that it just looked to be some bruising and told me to alternate hot and cold compresses and to call if there would be any changes or if I start a temperature. By that time, Bill and I were starving and getting exhausted.

We go over to Seasons Pizza for some lunch because I had an appointment with Dr. Warren for my balloon fill at 2:15 p.m. When we arrived, we were informed that she has been delayed due to surgery and that we can wait if we wanted to. Again, a long story short. HA-HA! We waited for more than an hour, but during this wait, Bill and I managed to get some laughter in and be patient. During my wait, we noticed a patient who must have just gotten her surgery and was getting her drains out. How did I know, you ask? Because I recognized the discomfort and the slow movement. She looked familiar to me, but I couldn't place her. When she was called back, her husband went with her, but her mom stayed in the reception area. I, of course, went over, introduced myself, and asked how her daughter was doing. During our conversation, I find out that she was around my same age and has two kids. The reason she looked familiar is that she is a nurse practitioner at my son's pediatrician's office. Her daughter came out. We introduced ourselves and exchanged information. I think this will be a lasting friendship between us. We didn't talk long because she needed to get home and I was called back. We got in to see Dr. Warren. She apologized for the wait and took a look. She said things were looking good and that we can fill them again today. So there we went with more needles—one to numb and one to fill. I got thirty more CC's in each and now was considered a B cup! Anyone who goes through this to get bigger is CRAZY! Be happy with what you have.

We made our appointment for the next fill and headed to the day care to pick up Zachary.

Now that my day from you-know-where is over, I am going to sit back and relax for the rest of the day/night.

OH, HAPPY DAY!

Monday, October 15, 2007

I was scheduled for my rescheduled MUGA scan at 9:00 a.m. I have been at little worked up about this so I ended up taking a Xanax just in case. But I don't like it. On the way there, it made me feel loopy and kind of dizzy. I don't know how my Mom can take them just to come see me for her dental appointments. Well, maybe that is why! We got there right on time, and the ladies remembered me. As I checked in, I got a phone call from Dr. Biggs's office, requesting another liver retest! How many times are they going to do a retest? So I told them that I would be over there after the MUGA scan. They brought me back, and I saw a different set of nurses. The one started looking, and it didn't look good. But she ended up feeling a good one. But unfortunately, it was on my knuckle! She said she hated to do it there, but it looked like a good one. She went in for the stick, and BINGO, she got it. Sure it hurt, but it was one stick, and it didn't burn when she put in the saline, which means we have found a vein! She injected me with the dye, I guess, and had me sit for fifteen minutes in the waiting room with the IV attached. This was so I wouldn't have to get stuck again. A man called me back and had me sit down on this table. They injected the radioactive goodies, and I lay down, while they pointed this X-ray-looking machine at the top of my chest. They started the test, and it went for about seven minutes. No big deal. People were walking back and forth, looking at the monitor, and then they come in to change the position to the left side. While they were doing this, they saw a radiolucency (dark area) on the monitor. They asked if I had a pacemaker, had any heart surgery, was wearing a necklace, etc. Answers to all were no, so they said it must just be an anomaly! After the test was completed, the nurse who did the IV was still curious as to what the dark area was, and she investigated and came to the conclusion that it was from the expander that I had in. They took out the IV, taped me up, and off we went to get another stick.

We headed over to the HGC and got the blood order. I saw Tawanna and asked if she could draw the blood. Out came Sharon, the other lady who has stuck me before, and I say okay and went back with her. Well, she tried in the crease and got nothing, so she got me in the WRIST! OUCH, THAT HURT! I am so not going to be a drug user!

Okay, that was done, and we were out of there. Later that night, the office called and said that the test came out okay and that we were still on for the first chemo treatment on Wednesday. Later in the night, I headed to the Cub Scouts event, which was nice because I was doing something other than visiting doctors.

Tuesday, October 16, 2007

My dad took me to therapy, and we went to lunch afterwards. Today, it was McDonalds, but this lunch was priceless. We sat there for one and a half hours, had a good heart-to-heart talk, and got a lot of "stuff" out in the open. You know, you never really get to have that one-on-one with your dad too much! I know I keep saying it, but family is AWESOME!

Later in the night, the calls started to come in to wish me luck for tomorrow. It will be my first day of chemo. After I put the kids to bed, I ended up reaching for Wendi's book and reading what she did the night before and the morning of her chemo. Bill and I held each other and fell off to sleep.

Wednesday, October 17, 2007

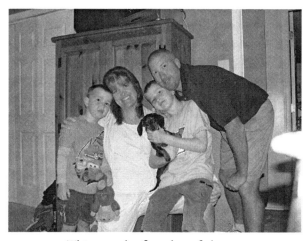

This was the first day of chemo

The day is here! We got a family picture before I went, and then we dropped Buddy off at our neighbors'. While we were leaving, I saw Joanne pulling down her driveway. I rolled down my window and waved to her since I knew that we needed to be there in time. Later, I found out that it was upsetting to Joanne, just knowing what I was up for. Okay, wipe the eyes, we have a Tx to go to. We dropped Zachary off at day care. Bill took him in because he knew that I would talk too much if I went in. We arrived and checked in. The nurse practitioner came in, examined me, and discussed the meds and side effects again. She also reviewed with us about all of the liver blood tests that I have had done. She showed me the numbers from the first test, which were sky-high. The second test showed that I didn't have hepatitis, and the third test showed that the numbers were much lower, but that I was in the gray zone for hepatitis, so they wanted to do another test. This did not mean that we couldn't do Tx; they just wanted to find out why the test was coming up that way. They would get this test from the port, thank goodness. She left the room, and Dr. Biggs came in, examined me, and discussed with me some of the similar topics. We left the room and went to the Tx room. I went, and the first thing you need to do is sign in. It was 8:55 a.m., and I let them know that I was there and ready for my first day! All of the nurses were very nice. Kay greeted us, reassured us, and told us that we could have a seat. We went and sat down, and Tracy came over, and she accessed the port. I was a little nervous since it was the first time that it was being used, but it was not too bad. She flushed it with saline and then drew the blood for the liver test. She flushed it again, placed some heparin (prevents blood clots), and taped me up! After she was done, she let me know that next time, I could get the shorter needle. Yeah! She then told me to go pick a recliner, and she would be right with me when the meds come up. Bill got me comfortable and went over to Wawa to get a bite to eat. So far, my nerves were fine, and all of the needles were over! At 9:55 a.m., I was still waiting for the meds. Finally, at 10:05 a.m., they administered the pre-med/anti-nausea meds. At 10:30 a.m., the nurse manually administered the Adriamycin (three syringes at a slow pace). They couldn't mix this and put it in an IV bag because it wouldn't stay mixed. This is the dreaded med that will take my hair and turn my pee pee orange for a day! Don't you just love the details! At 10:45 a.m., the Cytoxin drip started, and it would take about thirty minutes. She explained that I may feel tightness in my nose or sinus, and if so, they could slow it down. I did not feel anything, and I covered up with a blanket and got comfy. I had a slight headache from this morning. As I was sitting there, Bill was falling asleep, and I was thinking to myself, *I am sitting here getting chemo*!

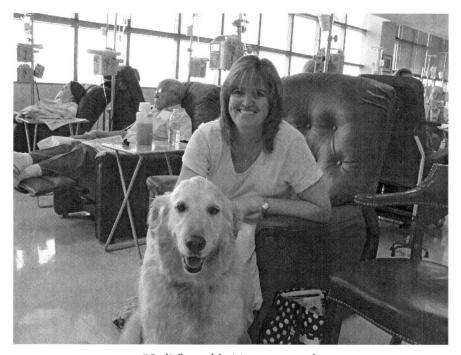

"Sadie" would visit once a week

During the Tx, I got to meet Sadie, the dog, who is a volunteer visiting dog. The drip was done, and they unhooked me. I got up to leave and felt fine. As I was leaving, I ran into my friend Kathy, the one whom I met at Dr. Warren's. She informed me that she had a tough decision to make. Her Tx is not cut and dry like mine; she has a lot of decisions to make and does not know which is the right one. It is a pretty detailed story, but the point to make is that you always think that you have the bad end of the stick, but sometimes, someone may have it worse. We were heading home, and I was making phone calls to my family. "Hi, it's me, and I am filled with CHEMO!"

Bill went to lie down. I was not tired so I got on the computer and typed up my update. Prior to sending it, I lost it! By the time I got tired, I couldn't sleep because it was time for the kids to come home. Lesson learned for the next time—even if I am not tired, try and lie down.

My family stopped by after work to check on me and to have some dinner. I felt hungry, but it was hard to eat. I got a banana and later ate some rice. It didn't taste good. Oh yeah, and I went potty, and it sure was peach in color! I made it through the day and now for my sleeping time.

Thursday, October 18, 2007

Bill and I went on a field trip to Milburn Orchards with Zachary. We drove separately in case I feel down. The day was good. I was a little tired and woozy, but I made it. We then headed home, and I took a nap when we got there. When I woke up I felt woozy and hungry so I took a couple of bites of Bill's sub. Oh that tastes good! I was able to eat a little better dinner, and I went to bed feeling pretty tired.

Friday, October 19, 2007

The kids went off to school, and I am resting for the day. I was hungry and knew that the doctor said that a lot of women gain weight during chemo. OH GREAT! So I got a Weight Watchers bagel and juice. But about two hours later, Sharon was still hungry. The time was ten thirty in the morning, and guess what she wants. The rest of the Sub from yesterday. So I went and ate the rest of the Sub, and it tasted soooo good. I felt like I have a hangover! I talked to Joanne, and I said how I felt was called my chemo hangover—my tummy churning, my feeling tired, and my need for greasy food. I know that the doctor said to watch out for acidic and greasy food during this time, but hey, if it gets me through it, I am there. That sounds to me like a good excuse to eat. I did make it to therapy today and rested the rest of the day and night. The kids are seeing how Mommy is unable to be herself and needs her rest. They are doing really well with all of this.

Saturday, October 20, 2007

I went to Buddy's game, feeling a little woozy, but I was hangin' in there. But guess what I had for breakfast. I had an english muffin with cheese and sausage sandwich. While I was there, I had hot chocolate and some soft pretzel with cheese. Buddy had a great game, and they played on the playground for a while as I sat in the truck. We got home, and I went to lie down while Bill and the kids played outside. Bill was exhausted but having fun with the boys. All in all for me, not a bad day!

Sunday, October, 21, 2007

HAPPY BIRTHDAY DAVE! My brother-in-law is in Iraq. He is safe and doing well. Please keep him in your prayers as well! This night, the reality of the hair loss is setting in. While I was talking to Buddy, he was saying things like, "Mommy, what am I going to do when your hair is gone? I won't be able to rub my fingers through it while you are reading to me!"

I told him that it is going to be very hard for Mommy too because I love when he does that, but it will grow back, and we can find other ways to relax. We, of course, get some joking in and start saying how I am going to look like a boy. Zachary said it would be okay, and he kept telling me that he is going to miss me when he is at school. The heart is hurting.

I went to bed, and Bill and I were talking. I told him how I am starting to feel reality setting in. That it is real—I have cancer and I am getting chemo. He was very positive and said that we are going to get through this. I know that I will, but this is a low point in my Tx. I did finally get to sleep that night.

Monday, October, 22, 2007

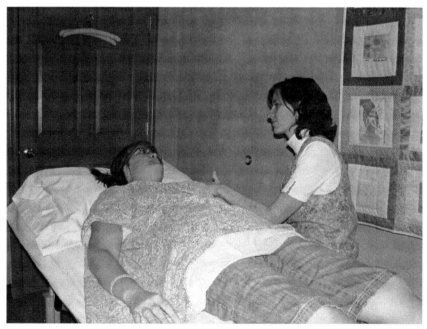

My therapy treatments at Specialty Rehabilitation with Lisa

I had therapy scheduled at 12:30 p.m. I got up, and the boys got ready for school. They were hugging and kissing me, and of course, I was still down from last night. They went off to school, and I was just sitting there, thinking to myself that it is time to talk to someone. And low and behold, my sister Joanne called, and I let her know how I was feeling. She reassured me, and I filled her in on what the boys have been saying. I also discussed how I don't see an end in sight—seven more Tx's, radiation, another surgery, hair loss, no energy, blah blah blah. I got off the phone with her and fixed my "normal" sandwich. I did some things on the computer, and I decided that I should go take a nap prior to therapy. Bill got home and took me to therapy. He couldn't wait to take pictures; he has done this all along the way. He also couldn't wait to go back with me in the room to see what she does with stretching. Not too exciting, but you know Bill. While we were back there, he totally told on me that I have been slacking on my stretches, and my spirits weren't too high today. Lisa told me that everyone has down moments, and it is okay to go and talk to someone. You would think this therapy is for mental therapy not physical therapy. I always tease her and tell her that she should get a double pay for her services with me. She also strongly suggested that I get out and do something fun. I was starting to feel a little better. We were done there, and off we went to meet Dr. H. I was planning on telling him that I want to be off until March 2008, and I was unsure of how he was going to take it. Once we got there, I was very happy and excited to see the girls. The spirits were high, and I was feeling it. We went back and talked with Dr. H, and I was very surprised at his reaction. He suggested that I come in a couple days for some help for the girls with the computer. I was sure that due to the time I had to be off, I was history, it's the business aspect of it. I didn't give any commitments as to when or how much I could come, and he understood. Our office has had a black cloud over it, but once I get back in there the skies are going to clear up, and they will never let me leave. Nothing like tootin' your own horn! Anyway, it was very revitalizing getting in there to see everyone and even some of my patients. When we left there, I was my normal self. I was back to positive Sharon. Nothing can bring me down now! That night, Bill took the boys to Cub Scouts, and I was home with Joanne, Jessica, Jaylyn, Joanne's sister-in-law, and her daughter. We had fun doing a little Cesar Milan on Darla (my miniature Dachshund) who has become very protective of me since my illness. Forewarning, don't be afraid of her. It's just that when you come to visit, watch your ankles. We are in the process of correcting that! I was feeling great tonight, and Joanne noticed that as well.

Tuesday, October 23, 2007

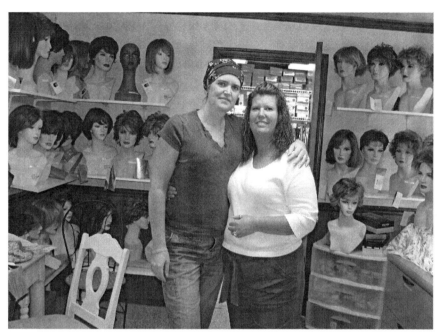

Lori and I at the wig shop

This was the day of "Mary." My friend Lori was taking me to Yellow Daffodils in West Chester for a wig. I know it is far, but my insurance covers this place, and I have heard good things about it. We got in there, and what an experience! She put this net on my head, and we started trying on different wigs—all colors and hairstyles. The lady showed us how to use the scarves, hats, headbands, etc. I tried on hairpiece bangs; you'd never know how much variety you have. We of course got plenty of pictures. Finally, we decided on "Mary." This wig is a short bob. It looks very nice on and has some awesome highlights. The lady forewarned me that I can't cook or go near flames or hot things because it could damage the hair! We got tips on caring for it, and $374 later, I was walking out a proud owner of a wig called Mary, a scarf, and a hat. Lori was a great help, and I was glad that she could be a part of it. We headed to Arby's for some lunch and chat.

Later, she was planning on giving me a short haircut and have the kids cut my hair. We get home around two in the afternoon, and I lay down for about two hours. We got dinner finished, and we waited for Lori. She divided the hair into four ponytails, and each of the kids got to cut one. Buddy really enjoyed it, and after this was done, he removed the ponytail and cut a little more. Needless to say, it made my haircut a little bit shorter than planned, but hey, it's only going to be there for another week or two. I informed Lori that I didn't care if I had a shorter spot in the back of my head; Buddy did it and he had fun doing it! The haircut was over, and Buddy blow-dried my hair and was having a blast!

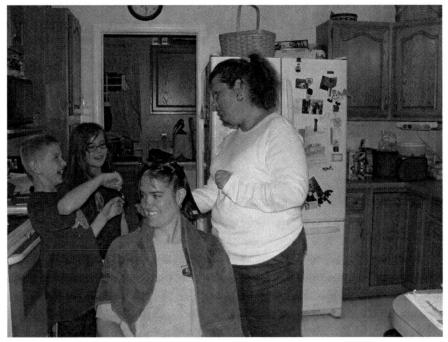

The kids helping me prepare for my hair loss

Scary thing was that when Joanne came in that night, we realized that the wig was so close to her hair style. Afterwards, the boys kept calling me Aunt Doe Doe. They liked it, and then they didn't. Zachary didn't want to touch my hair and then kept asking me to take it off! Before he went to bed, he said, "Mommy, your hair is short, and it is going to fall out because of the medicine; and then it will grow back, right?" Yes, he is only four.

Amazing! He said he loves me and that he likes my hair. Buddy kept saying he forgets about it and kept thinking I am Aunt Doe Doe.

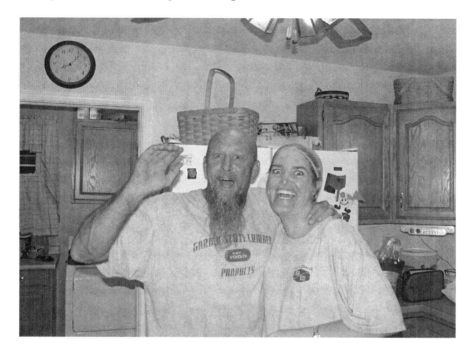

My neighbor Donnie and I having fun with the bald look

I had my neighbor Donnie come over to see my new hairdo and have some laughs. His wife passed away about four years ago of brain cancer. It was bringing back a lot of memories, but we are going to get him through this one together. Bill called and wanted to know how it looked and couldn't wait to see me in the morning. Time for night-night!

Wednesday, October 24, 2007

This day was just about therapy. Bill came home and liked the hairdo. I haven't had my hair short like this in a while, and you know what, it really makes me look like I have a skinny neck. Dad came over and took me to therapy. After therapy, which went very well, dad and I went to McDonalds for a little breakfast. We sat and had our little talk. He got updated, and then we left. On our way home, we took a little U-turn and went by our old house in St. Georges. We couldn't believe how run-down it looked. Not only our house, but the whole town. We then went to the cemetery and visited my grandparents' and aunt's graves and looked at old tombstones. I found out some history on my dad's family. We then went to the other side of St. Georges and did some sight-seeing and a history lesson of who used to live where. I tell you, the days with my dad have been the best. When would I have ever done these things with him?

I started writing my update, long as usual, but informative. I actually went and picked up Zachary by myself! Bill said it was like his child getting their license for the first time. He was nervous but let me go. I did fine, but I was still not one hundred percent comfortable with a long drive. We had dinner, and I took the kids to a book fair. I was feeling very good again and like my "normal" self. I have a week before my next Tx, and I hope that I feel this good for the remainder of the time. Oh yeah, I even went for a little walk around the development today (walking off all that sausage!).

As part of my update, this is what I wrote to everyone:

My experience so far has been okay. I continue to get cards, charms, and support from all of you, and again, I thank you! There shouldn't be long updates anymore since my doctor's visits are coming to a calm. It will just be the chemo and water-balloon fills, which I have tomorrow. I do hope that all of you enjoy your Halloween. Go carve a pumpkin, and while you are getting all the guts out of the inside, think of all of my cancer cells going into the trash! Go hug your family and appreciate your health!

I'm Back.

Thursday, October 25, 2007

I see Dr. Warren today at 12:45 p.m., and I think it will be for another fill. Since I had the morning with no doctors' appointments, I guess I will do some house-cleaning. Or not. Maybe I will just sit here and watch some TV.

Dad picked me up, and we headed to the doctor. I got my balloons filled with thirty more CC's of saline. It did not hurt as much today. Either I am getting used to it or it was a good day. Maybe I am becoming an addict. Yeah, right! I did ask the doctor how many more times do we need for the fills to go back to my starting size, and she said three to five. Not bad considering that I thought she was going to say six. After the fill, Dad and I went shopping. Surprised? I got a new vacuum cleaner. Who would think it is so hard to pick out a vacuum cleaner? It really isn't, but I am not good with decisions. Then we went to Wal-Mart, and what was supposed to be just to pickup of a couple things ended up to be more than that. While I was there, in the back of the store at the opposite end of the entrance, I started feeling a little weak and warm. I knew that I hadn't eaten and needed something to drink. Wouldn't you know they had a Subway there? So I asked Dad if he would like to get a bite to eat because I was getting hungry. He agreed, and we headed that way. I didn't tell him how I was really feeling, and well, my dad and I normally walk pretty slowly while we are shopping. And in this case, I was ready to go a little faster, but I didn't want to alarm him. It is so funny what we sometimes do to not make other people worry. Or, maybe not. What if I fainted prior to getting something to eat? That would have been worse than just telling my dad that I needed to go sit down. Learn from my mistakes, and just tell someone if you need something.

We made it to Subway and had a nice little lunch. Much better. I still never told my dad how I really felt. We finally made it home, and people continued to be jealous of our shopping adventures.

Friday, October 26, 2007

I was supposed to have a follow-up appointment with Dr. Clemmer today, but I called yesterday and cancelled it. She just wanted to do a quick check to make sure everything was okay and that I didn't have any more questions. So I would not see her again unless something happens.

Later in the morning, we got a phone call from the assistant principal telling us that Buddy has had a rough day today and that we needed to come and pick him up. He has been acting out and not listening to his teacher this past week, but today was a little worse. His teacher, Ms. Phillips, asked him to recheck his spelling words on the small chalkboard that he was holding, but he said that he didn't have to. His hand went up, and the board hit Ms. Phillips in the mouth, and she got a fat lip from it. This would have been grounds for suspension, but Ms. Phillips felt that it was not intentional. She did not want him suspended, so they decided to have him sent home to calm down. My boy is obviously not dealing with this very well. I think it is time to bring in the professionals. He didn't have a fun day at home, but we tried to talk to him about the situation. I called Pike Creek Psychological Center, explained what was going on, and got an appointment with Kym Champion. We have had to use her in the past with other family. She was great then, and I hope that she can help us out again.

I was supposed to have therapy, but I cancelled because I had to go to the school, and we have a busy weekend coming up. My sisters, the kids, and I were going to Chincoteague to my sister's trailer. Buddy and Bill were going on an overnight trip to the NJ Battleship with the Cub Scouts.

Sunday, October 28, 2007

We had a really nice weekend, had some rain, wind, but finally had some sun. We went into town, and Brenda had the kids do a "Build a Bear" for the trailer. It was relaxing, and we had plenty of laughs while we were there. We missed having Buddy there, but he had a great time with Bill doing the overnight at the NJ Battleship. I was glad that I didn't have to go when he told me about the tight quarters of the sleeping arrangements. He needed some one on one time with our "Budman".

Tuesday, October 30, 2007

I went to the doctor for my blood work and check. It shouldn't be a long process, but with me, that was not the case. I went and got the blood work and then sat in the reception area to wait for the results. They called me back, and I felt like I was at Weight Watchers. I got on the scale, and I have lost a pound! They asked me how I was feeling and what side effects I had from the first chemo. I did confess and let them know that I have not been using my baking soda rinses and that I do have sores in my mouth. The nurse practitioner looked in my mouth but was not concerned. Then she saw that I am from Middletown, and we started talking about Kelly's restaurant and Lester corn, and this conversation went on as if we were in a coffee shop or something. I bet you all thought that my process was long because there was bad news. Fooled you! Anyway, she asked me if I have gotten my wig because the hair should start to fall out after this Tx. I explained that it has been taken care of, but I couldn't find a wig with the grey patch right in the center like my hair! We laughed, and she looked at the clock and said she guesses she should be going. As she was walking out of the room, she said to Dr. Biggs, "Sorry, this patient just wouldn't stop talking!" She was joking, of course. Dr. Biggs then came in. I think it was nice that both doctors came in and checked me out. He was not concerned with the mouth either and told me to start doing the rinses. He then took his hand and was looking at where my gray patch is. I asked, "Are you looking at my grey hair?"

He said, "No, I was looking to see if any of the hair was falling out yet." Oops, my fault since we had just talked about the gray hair, I thought he was being smart and about to tease me about it. Okay, I feel dumb. Anyway, all is well and I am good to come back for my chemo. After my appointment, I had therapy, but it was not till 1:30 p.m., so guess what Dad and I did? We went to lunch. It was eleven in the morning, and there was no reason to go home and then come back out, so we would relax and eat at Season's Pizza.

Before I continue, I do have to tell you a story about the rinses. They suggested that I rinse with one teaspoon of baking soda with a glass of water four to six times a day. Well, guess what, I hate baking soda. I have been a bad girl and just figured that since I have been eating so many salty things, I was getting the salt that way. NOT! The sores in my mouth were from the crunchy foods that I have been eating. NOT. Anyway, while we were at the trailer, my sisters had looked in my mouth and said, "Would you face it and realize that you have sores and that you need to rinse!" They stopped and got baking soda that day and forced me to rinse. Of course, after I did it, it was not as bad as I thought it would be. Imagine that. To all of my dental hygienist friends, I was imagining the taste of the prophy jet. Now that is nasty! So of course, I thank my sisters for their persistence! I can't say that I am rinsing four to six times a day, but I am doing now more than I was.

Wednesday, October 31, 2007

Happy Halloween! It was chemo day for me. Joanne took me, and my friend Kathy was going to meet us there. I was hoping that Joanne would be okay! We had all our reading supplies like we were going to read. I signed in and went to sit down; they told me that I could go right to a recliner. My followers came with me, and we got comfortable next to a window. My nurse today was Dan, funny guy. The process was pretty much the same as last time. The difference was that we didn't stop talking/laughing the whole time. It was time for the Adriamycin, and Dan told me that by Saturday, my hair should be gone! As he was on the second syringe, I looked at Joanne and Kathy and said that my head felt like it was tingling. I bet my hair follicles were loosening as we spoke! Even though you may say, "Yeah right!" I really did feel some tingling in my head.

Anyway, my Tx. was over, and we had a lot of laughs while we were there. I was glad that Joanne was off from work and able to go with me one time so she could see that it was not that bad.

On our way home, we stopped at the grocery store to pick up a few things. Before we walked into the store, I did a test and ran my fingers through my hair to see if any was falling out. OH MY GOSH, there were about ten strands that came out! No kidding, it was happening already. Now, that is some strong chemo. We continued to go in and shop, but I couldn't stand myself, and I tried it again. Yep, there was more hair. Joanne asked me if I could stop doing that because it was making her sick. I, of course, was laughing the whole time. We called Bill and my mom to fill them in. I told Bill that I may need a barber; he told me to just say the word, and he would make the phone call. We went to check out, and when we got to the car, I told Joanne that I was feeling like my head was itchy, but I didn't want to scratch it. What if a big clump falls out? What if the wind blows, and it falls out? Oh, I couldn't stand it, so I called Bill. He made the call for the barber, and he was ready for me. We went home, unloaded the groceries, and got a bite to eat. I got the cameras ready, and Joanne asked, "Why do you want to tape or get pictures of this?" I told her it is a fact of life for me, and besides, when will I ever be in a barber shop getting my head shaved? NEVER, because I am not joining the army anytime soon.

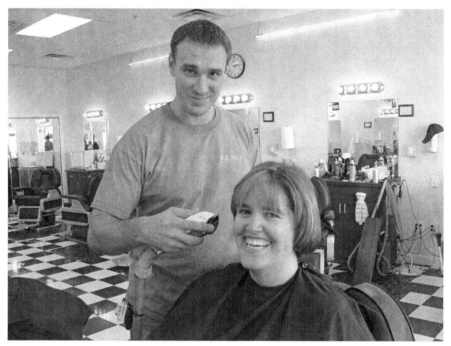

Tony from US Male giving me my new look

We headed on over to US Male on Route 40, and our friend Tony was all ready for us. I walked in and told him that I was joining the army! When I sat down, he asked me what I wanted, and I said, "You tell me."

He was a little nervous and said, "Oh no, this is all you." We finally decided to use a number one. You men, I'm sure, will understand that. I had to remind Joanne to get it on camera. During the whole process, I have to say I had a lot of fun with it! When he took the middle off and then the sides, I was more disappointed with how much grey hair I have! I looked like my dad; I guess that could be a good thing. My Dad is not bad-looking. Anyway, when I was shaved, I asked if he could put a message in the back of my head, like I love Bill. He thought that I was kidding, and I told him, "Hey I want to have fun with this!" Anyway, there was a guy there who shaved a ribbon onto the back of my head.

He then said, "Now, if we could do something with the caterpillars on the top of your eyes." No, he did not just call my eyebrows caterpillars! Well I guess they were kind of bushy! Don't worry; I did not get mad; I laughed with him. You know what; my head is not shaped badly at all! I think I look like GI Jane. Pretty sexy, huh! We were done there, and so I was off to get Buddy.

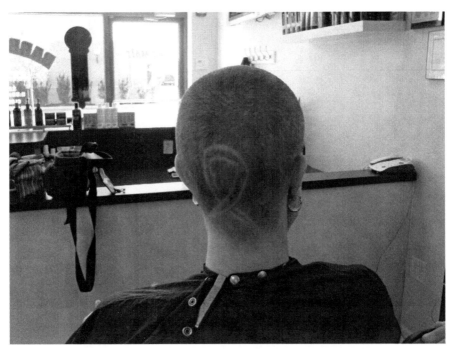

The artwork that was put on the back of my head,
you have to have fun somehow!

I did put on my wig because we had no idea that this was going to get done today, and the kids didn't know yet. As soon as Buddy saw me, he knew that I was wearing my wig. And then he told me to take it off because he wanted to see my hair. When I showed him my head, he called me a dude and said that everyone is going to think that Aunt Doe Doe and I are married, and I am the guy! He then told me to put the wig back on because I was embarrassing. I know that he really didn't mean embarrassing. No hard feelings.

We got to the psychologist. It was the first visit. I informed her about what has been happening, and she said that she was going to work on teaching

Buddy how to express his feelings and explain why he feels the way he does. Bill and I were also going to meet with her. Buddy went in and talked for a while. Kim said that all went well, and she would see him next week!

We picked Zachary up from day care, and he didn't have that much of a reaction when he saw my wig. His teachers said it looked nice but couldn't believe that my hair was gone already. When we got in the car, Zachary did ask me to take the wig off so that he could see my head. He thought the ribbon looked neat.

Then we were off to get dressed for Halloween. I was starting to feel tired, so the kids got dressed and went to Joanne's. They had to visit a friend of ours in Del City, and I decided to stay home and take a little break. My mom was there with me, and I had a little breakdown talking about my Budman and what he must be going through. I know that it will get worse before it gets better, but I told her I would go through chemo any day than to have him feel the way he must be feeling and not know what to do with those feelings.

Once they got finished trick-or-treating, everyone came back to the bedroom to empty out their bags and see what they got. They had a great time and didn't go overboard on too much candy. Brenda brought in the camera and took pictures of my new do! Well, this was one busy day, and I couldn't wait to hit the sack. I feel pretty good, just tired.

Thursday, November 1, 2007

I went to therapy, and the girls there liked the wig as well. But even if they didn't, do I really think that they would tell me?

Stretching was coming along and feeling good. I then went to get my Neulasta shot. I saw Dan and told him what happened about the hair. Some of the nurses came up to me and told me that the wig looked great and very real. Many say that my blue eyes seem to stick out more. I got poked, and then back home I went. This wasn't too busy of a day, and I am happy to say that Buddy had a good day as well.

Friday, November 2, 2007

I went to therapy in the morning and then came home and rested for the rest of the day. That night, my mom came over to sit with me while Bill and the boys went to a bonfire with the firehouse. As much as I would like to go, I don't think I would be a great company with the way that I was feeling. The boys understood and hoped that I feel better. They had a great time, and when they came home, Bill suggested that I spend the night at Mom and Dad's. That way, I could relax and not worry about the kids. I think that was a great idea, so I packed my bag and went home with Mom. I was tired and starting to get a little nauseated. It was also kind of nice sleeping in a different bed and atmosphere.

Saturday, November 3, and Sunday, November 4, 2007

We decided that I will stay the whole weekend at Mom and Dad's due to how I am feeling. I am pretty tired and pretty nauseated. Oh yeah, and I haven't gone poopy since Wednesday! It is very hard to get in a comfortable position. I sleep for about thirty minutes, and then I wake up and start all over again. The ache has returned in the back of my neck and jaw. I took a Correctol (ancient) because my Senokot was at home. My mom eventually went and got the Senakot for me to take. As far as the appetite, well again my "chemo hangover" has returned. I have that I-want-grease feeling, so at about four in the morning, I wanted to go out and get a leftover cheeseburger so bad. But I didn't want to wake my parents up as I knew my mom was sleeping very lightly while I am here. So I watched some TV and eventually went to sleep. When it was breakfast time, and my mom asked me what I would like. I told her my story and informed her that I still wanted that cheeseburger. She laughed and went to fix me my "breakfast." I don't know what it was, but grease seemed to help me. Talk about watching my weight.

I went home Sunday night, but I was not feeling any better. At this time last session, I was feeling a little better.

At midnight on Sunday, I took more Senokot. Watch out when this stuff works! I think I have every symptom all at once. I had a stuffy nose so I couldn't breathe through my nose, my belly hurt, haven't gone yet, couldn't get comfortable, and I was wide awake. I think I got about two hours of sleep the whole night! I was not feeling too good.

Monday, November 5, 2007

I got Bill up for work 4:10 a.m. and told him that I haven't slept and that I still felt crappy. I would be calling the doctor today. Bill was a little nervous about going to work, but I informed him that I would be okay and that Mom has taken off work and was coming over. I cancelled therapy (they were so understanding), and Mom got the boys off to school. She had a doctor's appt and then was coming back over to be my cleaning lady. THANK THE MAN ABOVE! My house was filthy, in a woman's eye. No offense, men.

Oh my gosh, I thought I felt something rumbling in the tummy! Oh yes, it finally happened. Not too much, but it was a start! Don't you just love the details?

The doctor's office called and said that everything sounded fine, but I had to keep taking my temperature. They were more concerned about the temperature and possible need of an antibiotic. But otherwise, all was good. Easy for them to say. I kept trying to get up, but I just didn't have the energy. And when I did get up, I felt nauseated again. So needless to say, as my mom was cleaning, I was just lying around; but it sure did smell clean!

Later that night, there was a "Look Good, Feel Better" class given at the HGC, and Brenda was planning on going with me. Bill would be going to Cub Scouts with the boys. I was not feeling one hundred percent fine, but better. Oh my gosh, before we left, I have gone again. Yeah!

We got to the class, and it was bigger then they had wanted. It consisted of all ages and all stages of treatment. Some women have already lost their hair, and some had their hair already growing back. They went over makeup hints—pretty new to me since the only thing that I wear is lipstick. They also have given us a whole bag of cosmetics. They went over some wig-care and some scarf demos. During the middle of the presentation, my tummy started rumbling, and I had to leave. I didn't tell Brenda, and while I was in the bathroom, she came in to check on me. She said that as she was sitting there, she thought, "Okay, she didn't even say where she was going. What if she passed out and I am just sitting here?"

I returned, and the night was almost over. They handed out handmade quilts from "Quilts of Comfort" that were donated. So nice. Oh my gosh, the tummy was cramping. Get out of the way, here I go again! I can say now that the Senokot was working. We finally got into the car, and I was feeling tired, no wonder. We stopped at Wawa to get me some Gatorade. Replenishment was needed! When I got home, I thanked Brenda for being with me. We laughed about our night. I changed into jammies, and I was ready for bed. I think I will actually be able to sleep tonight. Yeah.

Tuesday, November 6, 2007

I got the kids off to school, and I was feeling better but still a little tired. When I get up, I can't stay up for long periods of time because I feel shaky. You know, like you do when you have been down with the flu for a couple of days. Buddy had an appointment with Kym today at 4:30 p.m. He also had a half-day at school. I managed to take him to therapy, and it was like a click of a switch that I started feeling like myself again. The session went very well with Buddy, and he also had a lunch bunch at school today, which involves a group of kids who meet once a week. These kids all have a parent or sibling who is going through a sickness or chemo. He seemed to enjoy this.

As I was heading home, I remembered that there was a Ladies' Auxiliary meeting, and I felt like I need to go out and see people. I am very glad that I went, it was nice to see everyone, and everyone was happy to see me. I am feeling pretty good. Yeah.

Thursday, November 8, 2007

This was a very busy day for me, but I was feeling much better, and I have even gone to the bathroom without any help from meds! It was a proud moment. Anyway, I went to therapy and saw a big difference. Then I got the balloons filled again. I am getting bigger and harder. My girlfriend said it perfectly—it is like having a turtle shell on your chest. Doesn't that sound comfortable? Everything is healing nicely. Next, I was off to parent-teacher conference. Buddy is doing great educationally; he made it to the honor roll. Yeah! His teacher was not concerned and knew that he is a good kid and that we are going to work through his behavior. I then went and picked up some delicious chicken salad that my good friend made me, went to pick up Zach, and headed home and stayed for a couple of hours. Yep, I was feeling like myself again—on the go! I even drove today. After I rested for about one and a half hours, I got dressed because I have a Longaberger® home show to do! It was very nice seeing everyone and being able to do something. I have not felt weak or nauseated in two days. It was nice to be normal again. Oh yeah, and remember when I said that they informed me that I may go through early menopause? Well that has not happened yet, and boy is it a heavy one! I did, however, get a good night's sleep!

Friday, November 9, 2007

I got dressed, put on the wig, and headed off to a Continuing Education course for dental hygiene. Everyone was so happy to see me, and some even thought that the wig was my real hair! I felt good all day and came home with the boys to relax.

All in all everything is going well. My attitude is still on the up, and I continue to be thankful for all of the thoughts and prayers. My links of love charms are beautiful, and I still don't have any idea who started it, but whoever it is, I thank you very much! For those of you who do not know about the Links of Love charms that I keep mentioning, it is a bracelet that was mailed to me anonymously. I surprisingly received it in the mail one day with a letter, which was not signed, and a SS bracelet that had a starter breast cancer ribbon charm on it. After that, I would sporadically get a charm in the mail from family and friends that has special meaning with that person. It has been an awesome and sentimental gift to me. The funny thing is that when I received it I thought that the envelope had said Locks of Love and my response was, "Look they are sending me information about donating my hair and I haven't even had my first treatment!" Isn't that funny?

My next Tx is on Wednesday, so it will start all over again, but I will be ready with the Senokot this time!

Here I am again!

Saturday, November 10, 2007

The boys had a skating-rink birthday party to go to, but I stayed home due to the closed environment and all the kids. I did not want to take the chance of getting a worse cold. Oh yeah, I have a slight cold. It was Joanne and John's seventeenth anniversary, and they had a bonfire at their house. It was a beautiful night for everyone, and they had a great crowd. I, of course, did not wear my wig because I couldn't get it near a flame or hot stuff, or else I guess I would go up in flames! So I kept warm with my hat. I didn't stay out too long and then changed into my wrap, which, I must say, looked pretty good. Everyone again was very happy to see me, and I was very glad to be my normal self. My girlfriend Merith has thyroid cancer and has gotten a secondary infection in her eye which makes it lazy, so she was there with her pirate patch on. And we had a blast with our situations. She has a positive attitude just like me, and if she didn't in the past, she does now. I love her; she is definitely one true friend! Not to say that my other friends aren't.

Sunday, November 11, 2007

The boys had another skating party to go to, and I almost went, and then I talked myself out of it for the same reason. It was a beautiful day, and Bill, for those of you don't know, is a Christmas-light geek! He has gotten the setup where the lights play with the Christmas music, and you can hear it from your car radio when you pass by the house. So needless to say, he has been involved with that. He went to the party anyway. What a great guy. I stayed home and cleaned some, knowing I would be down by the end of this week. I was feeling pretty sore from the fill last week. I guess I am getting pretty close to my original size, and the stretch is getting tighter. Oh boy!

While I was sitting on the couch, resting, I just so happened to see if anymore hair was falling out, and I could just pull it right out and feel nothing. When Bill came home, he tried it, and so did the boys. It freaked them out because I couldn't feel it. I called my sister and asked her if she could put another design in my head by pulling it out, but she did not want to. I can't imagine if I still had my long hair. It WOULD be coming out in clumps. Gross!

Monday, November 12, 2007

When I woke up, I checked my pillow, and even though I sleep with a knitted or cotton cap, there were still little pieces of hair that I found on my pillow. I think the next time I am in the shower, I will try and really get the rest out. I don't want to see the patches missing; I would rather it be all gone. The kids are off of school, and they had their physicals. Buddy failed a hearing test in school and failed it at the doctor's office, so we were going to AI DuPont Children's Hospital for an official test. This was done last year, and he passed, but it was better to be safe than sorry. What more could my boy go through right now? We then went to the grocery store, and I came back and laid down while Bill worked more on the lights. I cooked dinner. Yeah! Bill had night work. He works overtime anytime he can. Thank goodness.

Tuesday, November 13, 2007

The kids were in school, and I had doctors' appointments. I went to therapy. I was pretty tight today, and Lisa felt it. I also find out that I have been a bad girl because I should be stretching three times a day and I have only been doing it once. Oops! I will try harder. I felt a little hungry, and I stopped and got a tuna Sub from Cappriotti's. It was really good! I then went to Dr. Biggs, got my blood work, and saw the doctor. My blood work came out fine, and I was good to go for my next treatment. I didn't do too good at "Weight Watchers" this week as I gained two pounds! I guess I should hold off on my Subs!

The nurse practitioner asked about mouth sores, and I told her that they have been small and come-and-go. She looked in my mouth and saw the one on the roof of my mouth. You know, the one that has been there. So she showed it to me and asked if I had been rinsing. I told her not as much as I should.

She asked, "Wouldn't that make you want to rinse more?"

I told her, "Not really, because it looks worse than it feels."

She said to try and rinse six to eight times a day, and I told her it is such a pain because I can't take a cup and rinse when I am out. And it takes so long to rinse a whole cupful. Well, she then informed me that I am making it harder on myself because all I have to do is a quick rinse, not a whole cup each time! So then I told her that I have been rinsing six to eight times a day because that is how many times it takes me to get through a whole cup.

She laughed and said, "Nice try!" So, needless to say, I will have a premix made up, have it next to the sink, and rinse more often. Dr. Biggs came in to check on me and said that there was a study stating that Taxol didn't have any effect on the type of breast caner that I had, but he doesn't feel confident enough for me not to get it. So unfortunately, I will be getting the four Txs of Taxol. Boo-hoo!

Later that night, I went to a Cub Scout training class at William Penn, and Bill stayed home with the kids. I went since I knew that I was feeling well, and I needed the training. Besides, after tomorrow, I would be back to feeling crappy. It was okay; you do what you have to do.

Wednesday, November 14, 2007

It was chemo day! My mom took a day of vacation to go with me. She was hinting around that she had some leftover vacation, and if I "needed" her to go, she could. Bill was off, but I think my mom just wanted to go with me. The ride there was exciting; I must say my mom doesn't do well with talking and driving at the same time. We did get there safely but with many laughs. Once we got there, we got comfortable and took our books again like we were really going to look through them. Al was our nurse today—nice guy and very talkative about what the treatments do. Mom was interested, but I have heard it before. This also limited us to our talking, but mom was being pretty nosey with what was going on around me that it seemed like the Tx was much shorter. We packed up and were on our way for my mom to get a blood test. She thought she was pregnant. HA-HA, just kidding. She did have to get a blood test though. When we were done, we stopped at Red Robin for a bite to eat. Nice place if you have never been there. A little on the expensive side. But if you are dieting, they will substitute a Boca burger for any of their burgers. Then we were full and tired, so back home we went. On the way home, I did notice that my salivary glands are on overload. I can't swallow fast enough when I am talking. The saliva just comes pouring out. The doctor said that increased eye and nose secretions are common, but leave it to me to be my mouth. So if I happen to drool (I don't know how to spell that word) while talking to you, I apologize.

I did come home and lie down for a little, but I think that hurt me more than anything. I wanted to go to a meeting at seven in the evening, and it took me a little longer to get motivated than I thought it would. Once I got up and moving, I was fine. I know that my mom didn't agree with it, but I have to keep on reminding her that I know my body, and when I can't do something, then I won't. Besides I have days coming up when I am not going to be able to do anything. UGH!

Thursday, November 15, 2007

Bill and I had our session with the psychiatrist, and it was a good meeting. We had some options to play with for Buddy, and we may consider some meds if we don't see any changes by the end of the year. Too early to tell right now. We then went for my Neulasta shot, and while we were there, I ran into a neighbor whom I didn't know, and she is going through lung cancer. It is a small world.

I will tell you again that the nursing staff at the HGC is so very nice; they certainly remember you after your first visit. Then off to therapy, I had some "cording" going on in my left arm, which basically involves a nerve that needs to be stretched. Ouch. But remember, no pain, no gain. By the end of the day, I was feeling tired, and I was ready for my nap. I got up for dinner, and Joanne had the kids for a little while. They came home, and we were in bed by eight in the evening. YES!

Friday, November 16, 2007

I was feeling off-and-on good, just no energy. Nausea comes and goes, and believe me, I am taking Senokot faithfully. I am waiting for the next two days to be rough, but I may go to dad's for a couple of days again. It makes it easier on Bill when he doesn't have to make sure that the kids are being quiet.

CELEBRATE!

Saturday, November 17, Sunday, November 18, and Monday, November 19, 2007

I stayed at my dad's. He was quite the host as my mom was in Chincoteague with my sister. It was relaxing, and I am happy to say that the nausea was not as bad. I kept up with the meds especially Senokot! My niece stayed with us as well on Sunday since she did not have school, and she wanted to be with Aunt Sharon. She took care of me while I was there. Bill had a very nice weekend with the boys and was getting some quality time with them. They understood why I was at Pop-Pops, and we talked everyday. My parents live ten minutes away from me, so it is not a very long distance. I came home later that Monday, and Bill was headed for night work. I was so relaxed that I failed to make Buddy's appointment for the psychiatrist. Oops! I guess we will just hang out at home tonight.

Tuesday, November 20, 2007

I was feeling blah today. No energy but determined to be better by this evening because I had to go to The Inn Keeper's Kitchen for a dinner that we won at a Continuing Education session. My hubby had to work, and my mom came over to watch the boys. I got dressed and put my wig on, which, I have to say, I don't seem to wear that much. I drove to my friends' houses, and then we all drove up together. It was so nice to get to see everyone, and the dinner was wonderful. The wine tasting was fun, but I do not like wine, Yuck! The place is affiliated with the Dilworthtown Inn. The night did grow a little too long for me. As we were driving home, I had a major hot flash, and nausea set in. We went on this back road, and the twists and turns started to really get to me. I couldn't get home fast enough. I did have to admit to my mom that it was a little too much for me, but again, it was a learning experience on how much I can do.

Wednesday, November 21, 2007

I had therapy, which went well, and then I went to Dr. Warren for my fill of the balloons. She told me that it might be my last one! She also said that if the scab from the dye is not off by the time we do radiation, then she will remove it and place the implants. I do hope that the scab comes off on its own because there is more chance of scar tissue forming around the implant during radiation if the implants are placed prior to treatment. Since my immune system is down, it, of course, is taking longer to heal.

Since Buddy and Jessica were off of school, I decided to take them to see "The Bee" movie. It is amazing that you can spend $50 just at the theatre. The funny thing is that while we were there, I ran into three friends, and they were all going to see the same movie. So it was nice to see everyone there as well.

I would like to let everyone know that I am getting through this, and at times, I can do some "normal" things. The movie was good, and the kids enjoyed it.

Thursday, November 22, 2007

Happy Thanksgiving! I was the lucky one who didn't have to do much, just heat up the ham. I relaxed pretty much all day and actually a little too much because we were supposed to be at my parents for dinner by four in the afternoon. We didn't get there until almost half past four. Dinner had already started, and I ate it, but unfortunately, my taste buds aren't back to normal so it was so-so for me. We went around afterwards and did share what we were all thankful for. We also started the tradition of making name cards and putting a special mark on one, and that person gets the centerpiece or whatever we decide for that year. Later that night, as we always do, we went to Ronny's Garden World to look at the trees, and the kids picked out an ornament. I didn't really have the energy, so I skipped it this year and stayed back at the house with my dad. I stayed and looked at the sale circulars for Black Friday, my favorite day of the season! That night, Joanne and I were undecided on what to do for the next morning. Mom didn't want to get up that early (four in the morning) to watch the kids, and Bill was working, and John was hunting. She did stay for the night in case she gets up and goes herself, but it just wouldn't be the same.

Friday, November 23, 2007

That morning, we had Mom come over around eight in the morning, and we went out. We did get a lot accomplished, and I only had to take one small break due to a hot flash. We went to lunch and headed for home. I can't wait for next year and hit the stores at four in the morning. However, as the kids are getting older, it is becoming harder to shop and more expensive.

Saturday, November 24, and Sunday, November 25, 2007

Not too much went on this weekend. I did know that this was the day when I wouldn't be GI Jane anymore. I was heading more toward Kojak. As I washed my hair, I have really been scrubbing because the hair was falling out. I continue to handle it well, but I do keep a cover on my head. It is amazing how chilly your head can get. I also wear it when the kids are around since they really don't like looking at their mom bald. Do you know how they say that you can get chemo brain? Well, it is kicking in on the forgetting area. Short-term memory is short.

Monday, November 26, 2007

I went to therapy, and I still had this "chording" going on in the left arm. It was frustrating to me. When I raise my arm, there is a "chord" that pulls and limits my movement. Lisa reassured me that it would work itself out and that I just need to stretch more! As if I was not doing it then. Well, okay, I could be doing it more. I then went to Dr. Biggs to get the blood work, and all was well. I unfortunately had to get the rear checked to make sure all was okay. I have had "diaper rash" from my eliminations, and they had to check to make sure there was no blood in the stool. That would not have been good, but all was okay. Later that day, Buddy had his appointment with Ms. Kym, and all was going well. He is handling himself well in school and working out his feelings. We then went to Cub Scouts, and the kids were doing well with seeing their den leader in a scarf.

Tuesday, November 27, 2007

The halfway point is here. HOORAY! I got my last treatment of Adriamycin and Cytoxin today. It went nice and smooth. Bill and I did a little shopping afterward and then headed home. He had night work, and so my sister came over to hang out for the evening.

Wednesday, November 28, 2007

I had another forgetful moment as I missed my therapy appointment today. Oops again! I got Dad to take me for my Neulasta shot but no lunch today due to lack of energy and appetite. Brenda came over with dinner tonight, and we watched some Christmas shows. The kids did fine, and dinner was very good, but I could feel the chemo setting in. Here goes another couple days.

Thursday, November 29, 2007

This was another uneventful day for me. Just laid around and relaxed. I did do some laundry and then laid down. I also received a phone call from Buddy's art teacher, stating that he and three other boys had been acting up; and the next step was a phone call to the parents. I did fill her in on what the family situation was and that he was seeing a psychiatrist and that he will get his hearing test done tomorrow. I also suggested that the counselor at school get involved and keep tabs on him. So, we will add this to the poor Budman's list. Mom dropped off some groceries and heated up some leftovers, and then we were left alone, and the kids were very good for me. Bud and I had a little talk about the incident in school, but it seemed like it was more just playing around then emotional.

Friday, November 30, 2007

It is hard to believe that it is the last day of November. Buddy had his ear test at A.I. today. Not that I hope they find something, but maybe that will answer some questions as to why we have to talk loudly and why the TV is so loud, and see if some of his school situations are related to hearing or not hearing.

I, as stated before, continue to take baby steps and try not to think of the long haul that still awaits me. All of the continued support and meals are much appreciated. My next chemo Tx is the Taxol, which will bring on a whole new set of side effects. I will take them as they come and hope for the best.

On the road again!

Saturday, December 1, 2007

Buddy's Cub Scouts were in the Middletown Christmas parade, and I was able to make it. I called my Uncle Kenny, who lives on the parade route, and I hung out with them. It was nice to see them, and of course, Debra was ready with the warm beverages. Yum, yum! Again, family is so great! Zachary didn't make the whole parade as it was pretty windy and cold today. So when he reached me, he stayed back and got warm with some hot chocolate and some hugs from me. Most people don't realize that you don't have any hair when you are all bundled up with a hat and scarf. It is when you get inside and you take those items off that you can just tell that people want to ask. I am very comfortable talking about it, but I know that some people are not. I was able to "hang" the whole time as I didn't have as much nausea this time. Of course it is because it was my last treatment of A/C.

Sunday, December 2, 2007

We put up the Christmas tree, and the kids had a blast. There were some branches with two and three ornaments, but that is what kids decorating is all about! That is why we have two trees, but this year, I don't think my tree is going to look that much better. I was feeling pretty good all day, but I needed to rest here and there.

Tuesday, December 4, 2007

I dropped Zachary off in the morning and went to therapy at 8:45 a.m. Lisa took some measurements and was happy with the range of motion. She said that we are going to work on that more. I had told her that I wasn't getting filled anymore, and she was excited—and I was too—that we won't be stepping back anymore! I left and went to Dr. Warren, and to my surprise, she asked me how I feel about the size. I told her, "I don't know. Are they the size when I started?" And she said she would like to do one more fill! Oh phooey, if she feels that we should, then I will agree with her. She reassured me that it would be my last fill. I am happy to say that I have about four hundred of more CC's of saline in these balloons. I am feeling the weight! She then went to tell me that she was going to trim some of the scab. She had to go and get the suture kit.

"WHAT! Are you going to cut me?"

"No, I just need an instrument that is in the suture kit."

As I was NOT looking at what she was doing, I could smell and feel the pressure of her cutting. How many of you have chills? As she was trimming, she informed me that she has had to cut more of the scab than she anticipated. The bottom part of the scab was open, and she was afraid of bacteria getting in and starting an infection. She removed some debris and then told me that basically I, have an open wound and that she wanted me to do a wet gauze (saline) and then cover it with a dry gauze. She wanted me to keep it moist and change it at least twice a day. The moistness will create new cells to form. Before she closes it, I asked for a mirror to see it. OH MY GOSH (I know that my girls from work can hear me saying this)! This is nasty-looking. She wasn't kidding that she had to take more away and that it was an open wound. In one area, I thought that my expander was exposed, but she told me that there was a thin layer of tissue covering it. She wanted to see me back in a week to check it. I was so grossed out and a little upset during this time. I called Bill to let him know what was going on and how I was feeling. He wants to leave work to be there for me, but I reassured him that I would be okay. I then called Brenda, filled her in on what happened, asked her to bring me some gauze, and asked if she would come and see it tonight. I was a little skeeved that I had to replace this dressing.

I told Buddy that I would come to his school and have lunch with him, and I was looking forward to it as I needed a hug from him. I had a good lunch and then ended up staying there for the remainder of the afternoon. It was nice to see how their day goes. It was also good to see how he acts, which is more of impulsiveness than misbehaving. He can't wait to say the answer before being called on. I felt some medication possibly happening! My mind was off of the wound, and the boys and I got ready to go to the firehouse for the Ladies' Auxiliary meeting. Before we went, Brenda stopped by, checked out the wound, and changed my dressing. It was easier than I thought, and she said it doesn't look as bad as I described it. (I think she was trying to make me feel better.) She said it looks like an ulcer that is trying to heal.

I left the meeting early to get the boys home, but as I went to find them, they were upstairs watching Rudolph with Daddy! Don't you just love all of the Christmas shows? Bill knew that we were down at the firehouse, so he stopped by on his way home from work. He has been worried about me all day and couldn't wait to give me a soft hug.

Wednesday, December 5, 2007

I had a rough night's sleep, a lot of coughing and sore throat, which has been happening. I took my temperature in the morning, and it was 100.3. Joanne took Zach to school, and I took Jaylyn to Nona's. I had to get an Rx filled, so I stopped by at Happy Harry's. It was going to take them thirty-five minutes to fill it, so I went to Dad's while waiting. He was still in bed. I think that he also has a cold. He said that he just didn't feel like getting out of bed. I updated him on what has been going on with me and how I have been feeling. It was a nice visit with Dad, and I told him that I was about to do the same as him. I picked up my Rx, went home, and laid on the couch all day. My temperature in the afternoon was 99.5. I think my cold was just getting to me. Of course, my mom and sister Joanne were nervous nellies because of my fever, but I informed them that I don't have to call unless my temperature is 102 . (For future reference, remember this statement.) I lay for the rest of the evening, and the kids and Bill allowed me to do this.

Thursday, December 6, 2007

Much better night, and I felt better. I took Zachary to preschool, and then I went to Buddy's class to volunteer again. It is amazing how thankful his teacher was for my being there. I wish more parents were able to volunteer in their kids' school. You really learn a lot about your kids and their education. I stayed there until two in the afternoon, picked up Zachary, and headed home. Not much happening this night.

Friday, December 7, 2007

Bill didn't have to work the overtime that he was scheduled for, so he took Zachary to school. I called the doctor and filled the assistant in on the slight fever the other day and the coughing and soar throat, etc. She said she would talk with the doctor and call back. The callback informed me that they wanted me to come in and get a blood test to check my levels. I was watching Jaylyn in the morning, and so we left at noon. We first went to Costco to look for tires for Bill's truck as they were pretty bald. To our surprise, he couldn't get the size of tires that he wanted because it was not recommended by the manufacturer. Bill got all ticked off because he couldn't believe that he has a big four-wheel-drive truck, and he is the only person who has little go-kart tires on his truck! As we were leaving, I could tell it was going to be a long afternoon. Long story short, no one would put on the bigger tires unless he gets new rims, which could cost one thousand to two thousand dollars. I said, "The truck is a 2003, why are you so worried about how the tires look now?"

He decided he was not going to spend the money on the tires when he is going to have to replace them in four years! Don't you think four years is a long time for tires? I know that some of you are bored with this conversation, but when Bill reads this, he will think about how silly he sounds. Think about it, you can't get bigger tires, so just get replacements and make the truck safe as opposed to leaving the bald ones on because you are mad and get into an accident and create more damage. Ladies, am I right? Thank you! Remember, don't sweat the small stuff or stuff that is out of your control. You know that I love you Bill!

Oh anyway, I went and got the blood test, which came out fine. But I told the doctor that my cough sounds like it is going to my chest, so he wanted to get a chest X-ray to double-check that nothing was brewing. During our conversation, I discuss the temperature (remember my statement?). He informed me that I am supposed to call when it gets to 100.5 NOT 102. The 102 was way higher and more dangerous. Oops! I wasn't even going to tell my sister and mom, but I couldn't resist. Besides it was 100.3 not 100.5. The chest X-ray was done, and they will call if an antibiotic is needed.

The afternoon was gone, and no shopping would be done like we had planned. I went home and laid down for a little while, and my mom has dropped off my bracelet with the charms attached. Every single one of the charms has such special meaning to me. Thank you to you all! I decided to go to the firehouse for a function. This was the first time I was going since my hair loss, and I didn't feel like wearing a wig tonight. I did well, and it was nice to get out and about. The boys did great, and Bill was able to get some time at the firehouse. So we all won!

Saturday, December 8, 2007

I was lazy in the morning, and as my sister came up for breakfast, I found out that she was pretty lazy today too. We finally got motivated to doing some things around our house. Bill took the boys to get their haircut, and I went to the grocery store for some things. Later that night, we went to the firehouse for the annual kids' Christmas party. The kids had a blast, and it was nice to see everyone. It was also nice to hear that I look good and that people enjoy the updates and wonder when the next one is coming out. It is like a TV series!

Sunday, December 9, 2007

Today, we were planning on making gingerbread houses and baking cookies—my mom, Joanne, Brenda, Buddy, Zachary, Jessica, Jaylyn, Gracey, Bill, and I. I started in the morning with chocolate chip cookies. Mom came over around half past ten in the morning, and everyone else showed up around noon. We do the cookie-baking every year, and this year, we added the gingerbread houses. I must say it was quite an event. It was Bill's and Brenda's first time making a gingerbread house, and it may be their last! Their house were the only two that didn't make it through the "storm." We had an awesome time, and we said that the adults are going to have a contest next year! We had spaghetti in the crock-pot, and we finally got finished cleaning up by seven in the evening. I feel like I did more lying than baking, but you know, you can't have too many cooks in the kitchen, right? It was a great day for all of us to be together, and everyone handled it very well!

Monday, December 10, 2007

I had no doctor's appointments today, so I went Christmas shopping and got some completed. I ran into a friend of mine from high school, and funny enough, we usually run into each other this time every year. During my shopping, I was starting to smell my "wound," and I felt like that meant infection. I have an appointment tomorrow, and I will get it checked out. We had Cub Scouts tonight, and we went to the firehouse for a fire-prevention lesson. All the kids had a great time!

Tuesday, December 11, 2007

Today was again another busy doctor day. I got my blood work and visited with Dr. Biggs. My levels were fine, but he said that I am becoming anemic and that he wanted me to start with an iron pill. Do you know what that means? Constipation, so Senokot, here I come! I also told him that my rear continues to be raw and that I am using baby-bottom ointment. He told me to get Anusol because that has some anesthetic in it. He checked my wound and smelled some infection (possibly superficial) and stated that if Dr. Warren doesn't give me an antibiotic, then he will (not being mean). He also reminded me to take my five Decadron pills tonight and then five more in the morning. This is to help prevent an allergic reaction. OH BOY! All is good, and he will see me tomorrow.

I then go to Simply You Boutique, and I bought myself some more hats/scarves to wear. Such a hard decision but much cheaper than paying to getting my hair cut and colored.

I next went to Dr. Warren's, and I let her know that I do not smell too good. She checked it out and didn't feel that there was infection going on. She said that the odor was coming from the other part of the scab, so she is going to remove that! She went and got the "suture" bag, and I saw her grab a blade. OH MY GOSH! Even though I don't have feeling there, I have a mental feeling, that it should hurt! She started by cleaning up the already open wound, and then she started picking and cutting. She could see me moving my feet and hands and asked me whether it hurt or if I just feel the pressure. I commented that I don't feel pain just pressure.

She said, "See, this is what it feels like when you are at the dentist, right!"

Anyway, the rest of the scab was removed, and she was happy with the new tissue that was forming underneath. Since I was going to be starting the Taxol tomorrow, and it would inhibit the healing process even more, she gave me an antibiotic ointment to put on the wound and an oral antibiotic as preventive. Of course, I asked for a mirror, and it looked gross, but not as bad as the first time. She wants me to apply it twice a day. I am not too sure about that, I am getting some phantom pain as I sit here and think about it.

I left and headed to Happy Harry's to get my list of meds. I've got my new scripts, my iron pills, my Senokot, and the good ole Preparation H (the generic of Anusol). Boy, did I feel like a mess walking out of there. As I got into my car, I felt this wetness on my shirt, and well, the antibiotic has leaked onto my shirt! Thank goodness I had something over my shirt. I looked like a mess, and I couldn't even have said that it was from nursing because it was much lower than where that leak would have happened! I tell you, there is never a dull moment. I finally got home, and the kids were coming home.

I fixed dinner; Joanne hung over till Bill got home, and then I headed off to some Cub Scout training. I got home at half past eight in the evening. Bill was putting the boys to bed, and I headed to the computer to fill all of you in on my happenings. I did take a break, and Bill helped me change my dressing. Not as bad as I thought since most of it gets absorbed or leaks onto my shirt (which I will have to remember for tomorrow). I was feeling nervous about taking a shower with the open wound, but I think it will be a good way to wash it off. Oh, but I am still nervous. What a baby I am!

Okay, so it is 11:20 p.m., and I need to get to bed. I have a long day tomorrow. By the time most of you read this, I should be sitting in my recliner with my feet propped up, getting my nice little cocktail of Taxol for four hours! My sister is going for a little while, and then my mom is coming up. Between the two of them, this should be a treat. They ask more questions about what it is, what it does, what the side effects are. I will probably sleep while they ask their questions. So if you are reading this between nine in the morning and one in the afternoon, raise your glass high and say, "Here, here, this is for Sharon!"

I will update you again as I take the next road of this journey. I am sort of, kind of halfway there and hangin' as strong as ever! You never know what life is going to throw at you, so just take every day as it comes. Thank you again for all of your support, thoughts, and prayers!

On a little side note, my very, very good friend Merith had some surgery last week (thyroid cancer), and I would appreciate any prayers for her for a speedy recovery. Merith, when you read this, I know that you can't talk that much, but know that I am thinking about you and love you very much!

HELLO TO YOU ALL!

Wednesday, December 12, 2007

My first Taxol treatment! I had to take five Decadron pills last night and five more this morning. This is to help prevent an allergic reaction. I am starting off a little nervous because if you have an allergic reaction to it, they give you oxygen, stop the Tx, and then start again. It sounds pretty serious.

Dan was my nurse, and he showed me this paper and said, "Now, here is a paper that we need you to fill out for any reactions, and you can see that it has not been used. We would like to keep it that way."

Joanne was with me in the beginning, and my mom was coming after she runs some errands. They started off with fifty milligrams of Benadryl, also a preventive for a reaction. This should make me pretty tired. As we were sitting there, my cousin Sue walked in. Joanne and I didn't even recognize her. I thought she was a patient just starting treatment since she had her hair and everything. We obviously weren't expecting her, but I was glad to see her. It has been one year since her chemo treatment, and she was caught a little off guard when she walked in. She told us that she became really anxious and didn't think she was going to make it over to where we were sitting before passing out. We gave her some water and got some crackers, and it helped her out. Of course, we were all laughing about it, but I know what she means about that feeling. Everytime I walk in to the treatment area and hear the beeping going on from the IVs, my stomach starts to turn. But then you talk to the nurses, and I calm down. Anyway, my mom stopped in, and Joanne was supposed to leave and finish some shopping. But she couldn't get herself to leave. I was feeling pretty tired. I ate some pretzels, and then I was wide awake. Gee, that Benadryl hit me hard, not!

They started the Taxol, and Dan had to sit with me for the first twenty min to make sure there was no reaction. The time went by with no event. Yeah! My brother-in-law, John, stopped in to see how I was doing. He has been so concerned with me during this whole journey, so I was glad that he came to see what happens during treatments. Pretty uneventful, which is a good thing, but curiosity can get you at times. Everyone but my mom left, and we sat there for the next couple of hours. During the end of the treatment, I had this coughing fit. I took two Halls candies and drank like crazy, and I was still coughing. It was getting on my nerves, and I was sure everyone else's. My treatment was done, and they unhooked me. It was about a quarter past one in the afternoon. My mom and I headed over to Cheeseburger in Paradise for the first time and grabbed some lunch. Not bad, but can you believe that I couldn't eat all of my lunch? I went home and waited for the kids to come home. Bill was on day work and will be home around seven in the evening. I feel okay tonight.

Thursday, December 13, 2007

I went to therapy in the morning, and I needed to pick up Zachary for his second series for the flu shot by two thirty in the afternoon. When I picked him up, he was not looking forward to the needle. But I explained to him that Mommy has to get one first, and he could watch me.

We went to the Helen Graham Center for my Neulasta shot. I was feeling okay so far. Zachary did very good watching me get my shot. We went over to the pediatrician's office, and he got his shot and did great. He was nervous because last time, he got four shots! We went home, and I noticed my jaw and neck pain starting to come on. It was early from the Neulasta shot, but maybe the Taxol was bringing it on sooner. Zachary showed off his Band-aid and was very proud that he got his shot without tears. I got my shower and headed off to bed. Bill took care of bedtime-reading with the boys.

Friday, December 14, 2007

We dropped off the kids to school, and Bill and I did some grocery shopping. We came home, put them away, grabbed some lunch, and I headed to Christopher's Salon for a pedicure and a manicure. It was a gift certificate from last Christmas. I explained my situation, and they told me that they could only extend it till December 31 of this year, so I figured I better use it. It was nice, but I got a student. She was nice but still needs a little more practice. I didn't get home until after four in the afternoon, and I have my office Christmas party tonight at Conley Wards Steakhouse. I got ready, and I was feeling tired and "bruised" on my back and arms. I used the bathroom, and I had blood in my stool. Of course, I called the doctor right away as they told me to, and I needed to wait for a call back. I got on my way to dinner with my cell on my side. I got to dinner, and everyone was happy to see me. They greeted me with hugs, and oh I was feeling the achiness (like a bruise) with every hug. During dinner, the doctor called back. He told me that it was not from the Taxol and to keep a check on it and that I may need to get my "tail feathers" checked.

Dinner was very good, but I was feeling a little strange, out of the loop, which happens when you haven't been to work in three months. Anyway, during the end of the night, I needed to excuse myself early due to feeling tired. As I was leaving, I got all emotional, but I got myself together by the time I was out the door. I was heading over to Brenda's for the weekend to relax after my treatment. She was looking forward to my coming. I got there about half past nine in the evening, and we stayed up until about one thirty in the morning watching TV, sitting by the fireplace, and talking. So even though I was tired during dinner, I was able to get comfy clothes on and lie down on a comfortable couch.

Saturday, December 15, 2007

Brenda and I had plans to go to Boscov's, but we never made it. We relaxed instead. Today, I was feeling some tingling, achiness in my legs, which can be normal. I took some Motrin, and it took it away. That was easy!

Brenda was getting Gracey today, and Joanne was having her spend the night, so they all came over. They brought some snacks and a smoothie for me, and then they were off. Brenda was going to a Christmas party and got me some movies to watch. She felt like she was being rude, but I reassured her that the reason I came up in the first place was to relax and do nothing. So the evening came, and the fireplace was burning. I watched three movies, falling asleep during the third one. The tingling continued to come and go, but I took Motrin, and it helped. Brenda came home safely. She asked me if I wanted to go sleep on the bed, but her couch was too comfortable.

Sunday, December 16, 2007

I had a nice night, and I planned on going home today. I watched some more movies. We ordered lunch, and as I was reaching for the menu, I noticed that my fingertips were numb! Oh, how weird, it is mostly my thumb and pointer finger, but the others are slightly affected. I headed home about three in the afternoon, and Bill was on night work, so I went to my Mom's for dinner. While I was there, my mom took care of the kids while I had to take a little nap on the couch. Numbness and just no energy! After my little nap, the boys and I headed home and got a good night's sleep.

Monday, December 17, 2007

Kids were off to school, and I was weak and numb (fingertips only). So I pretty much laid around all day. Later that night was Buddy's pack meeting/Christmas party with the Cub Scouts, and he was doing the flag ceremony. He did a great job, and they handed out awards and exchanged gifts, and then I was ready to go.

Tuesday, December 18, 2007

I had therapy at 1:30 p.m. I didn't feel like going, but I knew that I had to. I asked to ride the bike instead of walking on the treadmill due to my uneasiness. After the therapy was over, I was glad that I made myself go. I headed back home and pretty much did nothing for the rest of the day.

Wednesday, December 19, 2007

I took the kids to school and figured that I better get my shopping done. Well, I definitely could tell that I wasn't myself because I went to three stores, and I could tell you where every seat was. I just didn't have the energy to shop or walk. My sister kept telling me to give her a list, and she would finish it. But you know me; I was determined, and I knew when I needed to take a break.

I had to pick up Buddy from school for him to see Kym (psychologist), and while I was waiting on the couch, I fell asleep. So I guess that it is safe to say that the difference with this treatment than the last is that with the last one, I was nauseated and down for four days. With this treatment, I am not nauseated, but my legs are like Jello, and I am weak for a week and a half. Too early to say which one is harder. But we deal with it as it comes.

Thursday, December 20, 2007

This was not the best day for me. I had an appointment with Dr. Warren for her to check the healing. I have been applying the Silvadene twice a day like I have been told. Getting somewhat used to the look and the feel. My appointment was at 12:15 p.m., and Bill was with me (thank goodness).

When she wiped off the antibiotic and looked at it, she explained to us that my expander was exposed on the bottom portion—you know, the part that I initially thought was the expander when she removed the scab. I asked for a mirror, and oh my gosh, there was a lot exposed. I thought that it was a newly formed scab, NOT! She did not want it exposed due to possible infection, and we didn't want to loose the expander. I was not feeling too hot right about then. She explained that she was going to numb me up, deflate me some, and try to stitch the bottom skin to the "newly forming tissue," which was really not that strong, but we were going to try it. As she laid me back, I was thinking to myself I was going to get sick and faint! I am deflated 120 CC's of saline, and she stitched me. I didn't really feel anything but pressure. I just knew that she was suturing me. I think I almost broke Bill's fingers (we learned that you should only hold two fingers because if you hold three, you have the possibility of hurting the middle one). She finished and explained that some of the stitches may pop, and I shouldn't be alarmed. She wanted me to continue with the Silvadene twice a day and take another dose of Duricef. I asked for the mirror again, and it looked much better. No expander was showing. I looked like a mess, but I will deal with that later. No limitations, but I had to do light stretching. I had to obviously cancel my therapy appointment for today. I have mixed emotions—glad that she was trying to save the expander, but at the same time frustrated that reconstruction isn't as easy as it could be. But then again, that is my luck. Later that night, we went to Del City for a Christmas parade. I was feeling okay, but again, while I was waiting for the parade, I felt some leaking! When we got back to the firehouse to see Santa, Bill got me hooked up with some gauze and tape to take care of myself. I was feeling like maybe the doctor went through the expander, and that was where the leak was coming from. This would really be hard to do since the expander is so thick, but you know how your mind wanders. Bill stayed with the kids, and Joanne took me home. I got myself situated, and I couldn't believe how it was a constant drip. I will probably call in the morning.

Bill had written me this little note after one of my updates:

> *Hey, sweetie, it's your hubby. I am so inspired by you and your updates. I have wanted to tell you this in person, but either you or I am always too tired, so I will tell you via e-mail. I think you are the most fabulous person in the world. You have been through a lot so*

far, and your spirits are still very high. You are an inspiration to me as well as many other people. This whole process has taught me to be strong no matter how bad things can be. I strongly believe that for every minute of your life that you are sad, you are losing one minute of happiness. I am NOT glad you got cancer, but what I am glad of is that I am able to be with you every step of the process. I LOVE you so very much, and when this is all over, I know our relationship will be stronger than it has ever been before. Keep your spirits high, and I need to tell you again how much I LOVE you.

Love,
Your hubby

Isn't he just the sweetest man?

Merry Christmas and Happy New Year!

Friday, December 21, 2007

The leaking continued. I called Dr. Warren for her opinion, but I had to leave a message. I was going to the hair salon with Joanne to get my wig shaped up a little. Funny thing was that while the barber was cutting the wig, he pulled it off halfway. It was a funny moment! He shaped it some, but he was fitting me in and wanted me to come back so he could shape it up more. But I don't wear it that often. Anyway, it looks better. While I was there, Dr. Warren returned my call and informed me that it was just my body knowing that something had been done to it, and it was releasing body fluids just like it did after the initial surgery with the drains. She reassured me that it was not the expander that was leaking. We ended up doing some Christmas shopping after the hair appointments. I was very self-conscious about my leaking and was constantly checking myself. At night, I just relaxed with the boys.

Saturday, December 22, 2007

When I got up, I went and laid down in the living room. While I was lying there, I felt a little pop, and I thought that it was a suture that just popped. I went to change my dressing, and I called Bill immediately and asked him if that was my expander showing. And lo and behold, it was. I was not too happy, but Bill reassured me that Dr. Warren said that some of them may not hold. I tried not to think too much of it since we had a busy day and night. We had a skating party to go to for Buddy's friend, and Brenda watched Zachary. Later at night, we had Santa coming to visit at Joanne's house. (We have done this for maybe six years for the kids.) Everyone had a great time, and it is always nice being with your family. I, of course, was still thinking of my expander being exposed, but I did have a good time.

Sunday, December 23, 2007

Nothing really went on aside from me relaxing. It was a gloomy rainy day. We were supposed to go Christmas caroling tonight with the firehouse gang, but it was cancelled due to the weather. Unfortunately, more, if not all, of the stitches have come apart. I was having a down day, and I was blaming myself for not taking it easy with the stitches. I was going back to regular activity and doing light stretches, but I felt that I should have watched the lifting and other activities more. I ended up calling the doctor on-call, and when she returned the call, she basically told me that I could continue to put the Silvadene on and wait for Dr. Warren. Or I could come in, and she could remove the expander, and I could pack it twice a day. WHAT! I think I will stick with option number one. She had said that because Dr. Warren had sutured it once and that she (on-call doctor) wouldn't try to suture it up again. Okay, that didn't sound like good news. When I got off the phone with her, I was not too high-spirited. And then Brenda called me, and I had a breakdown. She reassured me that it was not my fault and told me to stop blaming myself. I have not had much good luck during this process, and this was just another bump in the road. She had a good talk with me, and as much as I could, I felt a little better. At the dinner table, I broke down again, and Buddy asked me, "What's wrong, Mommy, why are you crying?"

I tell him that Mommy is just a little upset and that this is hard to go through and that I am trying the best I can. He said to me, "I think you are doing a great job!"

More tears, of course. But you know, when you have a nice cry every now and then, it really makes you feel better.

Bill was on night work, so I filled him in when he called. It is hurting him that he can't be with me, but I reassured him that I was doing better and would be fine until he gets home. These kinds of times are when Bill can not stand work, but then again who wouldn't?

Monday, December 24, 2007

On Christmas Eve, we went to my parents' house for dinner—usually lasagna and buffet-style. Brenda wanted me to come over early so that she could do my makeup. As most of you know, Sharon doesn't wear much makeup, but it did look nice—not too much. You remember the "caterpillar" eyebrows? Well, they definitely are not caterpillars anymore. Very thin brows, if any, runs near the top towards the middle. An eyebrow pencil is hard to use if you are not makeup-savvy. We had another good evening. Unfortunately, Bill was on night work. With a full belly, we headed home and got ready for the big man to stop by. The kids had on their Christmas jammies from Aunt Brenda. We read "'Twas the Night Before Christmas," and the boys choose to sleep in the doorways of their rooms. This way, when Santa comes, they could see him! As I lay in bed, I remembered my nights before Christmas as a kid and then looked at my kids. They were so cute lying there. Life is good!

Tuesday, December 25, 2007

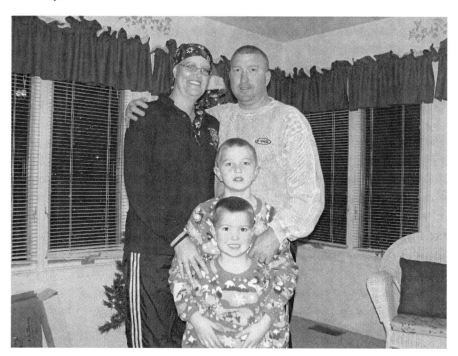

Family photo at my parents house

Merry Christmas! We had a great day, and I tried to forget all about my cancer endeavor for the day. Santa didn't go overboard this year, and it was eventful. Bill was home by seven in the morning and got everything ready.

Even though the leaking continued, it did not put a damper on our day. We opened our gifts, put toys together, and played with toys. Bill always makes Christmas breakfast, and I get clean-up duty. My mom and dad came over and saw what everyone got. While they were here, Joanne and her family walked up in their jammies and visited. We then went to her house and saw what they got.

We later went home and got ready to go to my sister-in-law's to exchange gifts and visit. We always enjoy that time because of all of the reminiscing that Bill and his sister do when they were kids. You would think that we would go home after that, but we then headed to my parents' again and had dinner and basically had another Christmas. We all love getting together and celebrating this time. The kids' favorite part is finding the pickle in the tree. We have an adult find and then a kid find. My parents have kept track of who has won each year, so it is pretty competitive, but fun. After all is said and done, we packed up the cars and headed home. Everyone has had an awesome time together, and I was feeling the love that my family has for one another!

Wednesday, December 26, 2007

Even though it was the holidays, there was no time to waste for treatment. I was able to enjoy the beginning of the day, but then I had my blood work and doctor's visit in the afternoon. My appointment was at 3:20 p.m., and I never left there until 5:20 p.m. Due to the holidays, being double-booked and covering for another doctor made them a little behind. Working in a dental office and being on the other side, I know it really makes a difference to let the patient know if the doctor or whoever is running behind, which I was not told. I only found that out from an unhappy patient who had been waiting and went up to the receptionist to find out what the problem was.

Anyway, when Dr. Biggs looked at the open expander, which looked like it was protruding at that point, he was not too sure if I will have chemo tomorrow. I informed him that I will be seeing Dr. Warren in the morning prior to chemo. He wanted to see me when I am done with her and then we would decide. At night, I was at Joanne's for movie and popcorn night, but while I was there, I felt the need to call Dr. Warren. At my last visit, she told me to come in on Thursday only if I needed to. Well, I think that I need to. In the beginning of my treatments, she had given me her cell number, and I felt uncomfortable calling, but I thought

116

it would be nice for her to know what was going on before I got there. She did answer, and I caught her by surprise, but she was okay with me calling. She told me to come in, and she would take a look at it, and we would possibly suture it up again. I told her that my biggest fear is losing my expander, and she said, "Well, of course it is, but let me take a look before we think of that." When I got off the phone with her, I felt a sense of relief. She, as I have said, is like my angel that is looking after me. She is GREAT!

Thursday, December 26, 2007

My mom was planning on going to chemo with me, but since I had to go Dr. Warren first, Brenda was going to go with me. My mom couldn't handle the expander part, and Brenda could be my second set of listening ears. This was a big thing to remember when you know that you are going to get some important information.

Dr. Warren took a look at it and said, "Oh yeah, all of the sutures are ripped, and the expander is exposed again. But the top part of the wound is forming good granulation tissue."

She suggested that she takes another one hundred twenty CC's of saline out and that we try to suture it up again but more to the stronger granulation tissue. She put more and stronger stitches in and told me to switch from silvadene to Bacitracin twice a day. She told me not to do jumping jacks, and believe me, I will be very careful this time. She wanted to see me next week to check things out. Brenda asked what we were ultimately trying to accomplish, and Dr. Warren stated that we want a new tissue to form so we can do the expansion again. We are now working against time because we need the skin to form. Expansion is done prior to radiation because radiation reduces the elasticity of your skin, which, in turn, will make it harder for the expansion. So please pray for my quick healing I headed over to Dr. Biggs, and when he saw the stitching, he said that he didn't want to do the chemo today because he wanted me to get a week's worth of healing. Since the chemo slows down your healing process. He said it would not put a damper the results and would be better for me. I was a little down because it put me back a week, but after further thought, I realized again that things happen for a reason, and it is for the better. I get to feel good an extra week, which includes my birthday! I also get to be with my good friend who will be getting her first chemo Tx and be there for support for her. So it is all good!

—

Mom and I hit the grocery store and headed home. Even though I didn't do too much today, I was ready to go home and relax.

Friday, Saturday, and Sunday—Can't remember too much what went on, but I put away some presents and cleaned the house while I have the energy.

Monday, December 31, 2007

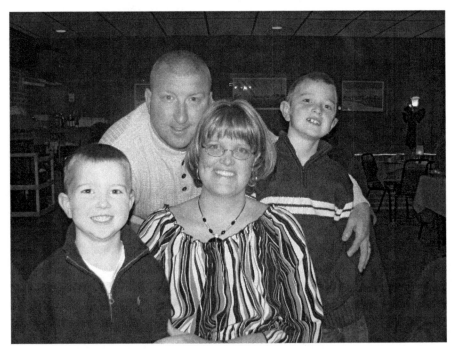

Dinner at Wesleys; like the wig?

Happy Birthday to me! I had therapy at 9 a.m., and they were careful with me. They could tell that I was nervous about having my suture reopened, so my visit was on the shorter side. I then went and bought a new outfit for dinner tonight and picked up some last-minute treats and drinks for tonight. We normally have people over at our house and bring in the New Year with all the kids, family, and friends, but this year, we had planned on me being pretty much under the weather, so we went low-key. My family went to dinner at the Wesley Steakhouse, which was okay. We used to go there when we were kids for my parents' anniversary, so it has been a while since we have been there. I had a cake that was sent to me and our friend Stacey, whose birthday is on the first of January. We all left to get into some comfy clothes and we met back at my house, hung out, played games, and brought in the New Year safely. We had some sleepover guests, and we finally got to bed by two thirty in the morning.

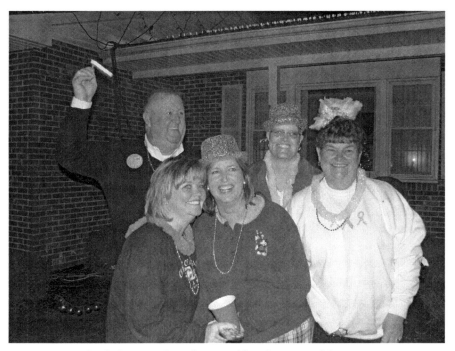

Dad, Joanne, Brenda, myself and Mom celebrating
New Years Eve/my birthday

Tuesday, January 1, 2008

It was late morning, but we had breakfast, and then we headed down to Middletown for the Hummers Parade. This is a funny parade of the happenings from the year 2007. Some of my family was there, and they were glad to see me. The wound seems to be healing well, no sutures have opened, and I am very hopeful.

Wednesday, January 2, 2008

Today was another full day of doctors' visits. First, I saw Dr. Warren, and she was very happy with what she saw. More tissue growth was starting to happen, and she wanted to see me in two weeks because she may remove some of the stitches. I then went to therapy, and again, it was on the lighter side. We continued to stretch as much as we could. The doctor may put me on hold during the radiation Tx, but we'll decide when the time comes. Next, I went to get blood work and saw Dr. Biggs. He was happy with the blood work and said that we are okay to do chemo tomorrow. My niece and Buddy were with me today because they had no school. They were great, and Jessica and I went to get our nails done while Buddy played Daddy's Sony PSP. We came home, got dinner, and headed off to wrestling practice. Both boys were trying out this season. What a treat to watch them.

Thursday, January 3, 2008

Chemo day. This is my second Taxol treatment. I was going to go by myself, but Mom didn't want me to go alone. Joanne said, "What if you have a reaction, and you are there by yourself?"

So my dad planned on going with me. Zachary was in school, Buddy was at his friend's house, and Bill was working. My appointment was later than usual—12:20 p.m. I got settled in. They put the Benadryl in, then saline, and then they started the Taxol. Twenty minutes into the Tx, I started sneezing, like fifteen times. I grabbed a tissue, and it still continued. So I went to the bathroom and looked in the mirror and noticed that my nose was all red, and it looked like I have had a reverse brow waxing. My brows were all red in the middle. So as I left the bathroom, I noticed that my third knuckle and the area around my wrist was all red. I informed the nurse, Julie, and she brought over Dana. They stopped the Taxol, started saline, and went to get Dr. Biggs. Thank goodness they didn't put it over the intercom because a whole group of doctors and nurses would have come. My fingers were tingling, like how they feel when they are waking up and more hives are starting. As we were waiting for Dr. Biggs, my dad laughed because I asked him if he noticed how red I was turning. But he said he just thought I had rubbed my eyes. Also, I remembered the first Taxol treatment that I had and the coughing spell that I had. Gee, I wonder what will happen during the next treatment. Dr. Biggs arrived, and he informed them to give me a shot of Decadron and wait twenty minutes. He came back to check on me, and the hives have gone away. They started the drip at a slower pace and continued to check my blood pressure and pulse oxygen. All of the nurses were great and continued to check on me. Of course, with my sense of humor, we got through it. I did not have any throat closure, which was a good thing. I definitely would rather have this reaction. The drip continued, and no more hives or reactions happened. My dad and I commented on how thankful we were that Joanne or my mom weren't with me during this Tx. They would have needed medication! Joanne of course rubbed it in, saying, "See, it is a good thing that someone was with you." But even if they weren't, it wasn't that severe of a reaction. I was calm and got through it. We closed up shop. We were the last ones to leave at around a quarter past five in the afternoon. While I was there, a lady in her late forties was there for her first Tx, and she was very upset, crying and all. So I, of course, went over, talked with her, shared my experience, and reassured her that she would be okay. She was very thankful and appreciative of me talking with her, and we exchanged information. The nurses even thanked me for doing that. Is this something new? Don't people help others? But then again, you know me, I will talk to anybody.

My mom met us at home and had dinner waiting for us. We had a relaxing evening. The kids were playing, and Bill was on night work. At about nine thirty in the evening, my hands started to itch really bad. I put an ice pack on it, and it calmed down some. Then I went to bed, fell asleep, and woke up around 12:50 a.m. with my body itching all over. I made a phone call to the on-call doctor. He called back very quickly and told me to take some Benadryl every six hours. I did that and the itching was taken away in twenty minutes! I slept the rest of the night.

GOOD NEWS!

Friday, January 4, 2008

I woke up and took more Benadryl. No more itching. No symptoms as of yet, but believe me, I will keep you informed if anything does. Bill is off this weekend and will keep the kids preoccupied. I went to get my Neulasta shot later today, and now I'm just waiting for the bruising to come.

So far, this is my life in a nutshell, and more adventure continues. I must say it is always something in me, but somehow I get through it. I have my family and friends to thank for this. I try to keep my life as "normal" as I can, and that is what keeps me going. It is hard not to do the things that I normally do, but I know that I will get there soon enough.

Saturday, January 5, 2008

I didn't do too much today. Bill was taking down some of his Christmas lights and going to sign the boys up for baseball. Later at night, Bill and I had the Fireman's Award Banquet at the firehouse. I was feeling okay to go. Joanne watched the kids, and we headed to the event. Everyone was very happy to see me and said that I looked good. I, of course, was feeling all bruised again, and the hugs were tough. But I got through it. We actually were able to stay until about midnight. I didn't do the dancing that I normally do, but they will be ready for me next year, especially my good friend Jay.

Sunday, January 6, 2008

This was a recoup day for me and should have been for Bill, but as long as he kept on moving and taking down more lights, he was good to go. Bruising feeling was not as bad, and I continued to take Motrin to help out.

Monday, January 7, 2008

Believe it or not, I had no appointments today. So I did a little bit of nothing. I was a little achy, and the numbness was starting in the fingers and the feet, but nothing too bad. Yeah! I undecorated my tree upstairs, and Bill will take it down and store it. But as most of you know, I will be sitting right next to him to make sure it is packed the right way. My items usually always fit in their original boxes. Some people call this an illness.

The boys had wrestling practice tonight, but Bill was home with enough time to take them. Their practice was for two hours. I don't have to do much but sit there. But I thought it was better if I stay home.

Tuesday, January 8, 2008

Even though I am not getting the "true" physical therapy, they still want me to come and exercise. They told me that I can do it at home, but I think they know me pretty well. If I don't go, I won't do it. So, I went there at nine thirty in the morning, and it did feel good to go once I was there.

This was a pretty uneventful day for me. We went to cub scouts at seven in the evening, and then the night was over.

Wednesday, January 9, 2008

I was invited to join my workmates for lunch and sit in on their staff meeting. I was able to stay the whole time, and it was great being in there and knowing that I hadn't forgotten how to do some things. It was also nice to see what is going on in the office while I have been out. I do miss being there, but I definitely do not miss getting off at five in the afternoon and running into traffic and then rushing to do the evening activities. Getting off at four sounds like a really good idea to me!

The boys had wrestling practice at six in the evening, so I stayed there for an hour, and Bill showed up after work. I had to go to a committee meeting for Cub Scouts, which was in the development next to where the practice was. So off I went to the meeting. I tell you, nothing is going to keep me down too long. It is great to have involvement in your kids' activities. Especially when they enjoy it and they are not being pushed to do it. Enjoy every minute that you can.

Thursday, January 10, 2008

It was another therapy day, and that is about it. I came home, and I did a little bit of cleaning, but I can't do too much for too long, because I get tired quickly. I get the feeling that I need to sit down after being up for a while. No nausea, just weakness. Later at night, Bill did put the tree away, and he did very well. He didn't get frustrated and it fit perfectly. Later on, he informed me that he did get frustrated, but he held it in! He is such a good man.

Friday, January 11, 2008

I ran some errands, did some cleaning, and was getting ready for my night away with my mom and sisters. My mom got tickets to see "Elvis" in Lancaster PA at the American Music Theater. My sisters and I were so excited, little sarcasm there. I said, "See you later," and gave kisses to the boys and Bill. *Here is a little side note, I have to tell you that I try not to say "goodbye" but "see you later" instead because "goodbye" seems so permanent. The funny thing is that I didn't just start this since my cancer diagnosis, I have always done this. Kind of weird, huh?*

Anyway, we listened to Elvis the whole way up there to get in the "mood." We checked in to our room and then went to Ruby Tuesdays for dinner. We didn't waste any time to get something to eat. Actually, we couldn't because the show would start soon. We got to the theater, and our seats were the very last ones up top, and they still were a good view. There was a young "Elvis" and an older "Elvis." Mom liked the older one better, and guess what we were trying to figure out the whole time? We wanted to know if he was wearing anything under that white suit. There were no lines anywhere. We concluded at a close-up view during autograph session, and with Joanne taking pictures, that it was a G—string he was wearing. Or it was built in to his outfit. We had a great time, and it was better than expected. I didn't wear my wig, but I did wear a "scarf" with a really sharp-looking hat that my sister gave me for Christmas. I felt good.

We went back to the room around eleven thirty in the evening and called it a night. I must say that during treatment, I do pass some gas, and it is usually in the evening and in close quarters. It is sometimes hard to hide it. So needless to say, we needed a candle but had to use baby powder spray instead. Hey, if you ever have to go through this, you will know what to expect. Side note, have matches with you at all times!

Saturday, January 12, 2008

We slept in and checked out at eleven in the morning. We went to Cracker Barrel for lunch and then headed off to do some shopping. I was doing okay, but like before, I did feel the need to sit down occasionally due to weakness. Of course, Mom was right there watching over me to make sure I was okay. We had a very long day of shopping, but we had a great time and got some good deals. We ended up at the Sonic drive-in for dinner. This is where they drive up to your car on roller blades. We then headed home. I passed out and fell asleep for a little while, and we got home around seven in the evening. When I got home, I went straight to bed. I felt pretty achy and had to take some Tylenol PM. The boys were in bed, so I will see them in the morning.

Sunday, January 13, 2008

This was just another recoup day, and I took the decorations off of the downstairs tree and put it away. When I was done, I went to take a shower, and I noticed a "bubble" on my wound. I didn't pop it, yeah, right; but when I was wiping it off, it popped, and all of this fluid squirted out. The bubble was all gone, and I proceeded to get a shower. When I got out, I checked out the situation. When I pump my arm, fluid comes out, and when I take a deep breath, more comes out. I figured that I should stop playing and cover it up, but I felt like I did too much; and I went to sit on the couch for the rest of the day.

I have an appointment with Dr. Warren tomorrow, so I am not too worried about making a phone call. We went to Joanne's for dinner, and Bill had a meeting for Relay for Life. We are thinking of having a Beef-and-Beer as a fundraiser for the event, but we have to put more thought into it.

Monday, January 14, 2008

I went to Dr. Warren, and she was very happy with the progress. She had to remove some of the stitches because they were loose from the swelling that went down (that I didn't know I had). She explains that the "bubble" was a protein layer, and it is like a blister, but nothing harmful. She then put more stitches in and really closed up the open area. So now, it is sutured skin to skin over three-fourths of the area. She doesn't need to see me back for two weeks, and she hopes for more healing! I had a therapy appointment afterwards, but I cancelled it so that I don't reopen anything. I am being very careful with this area; I really don't want anything else to happen. Since I was out, I went to get my tire checked for a slow leak, and of course, they couldn't plug it because it was too close to the outside wall. We have to get a new one! After they put on the new tire, and I paid the "cheap" bill. I went grocery shopping, and the numbness was starting to wear off. I was feeling a little soreness when I push the cart, so I compromised and did it with my foot and by sliding it. People were probably wondering what was wrong with me. Didn't I just say I was going to be careful with this area?

I picked up Zachary from day care. Buddy did his homework. We had dinner and then went off to wrestling practice.

Tuesday, January 15, 2008

When I woke up, I checked the area, and all looked to be holding. So I covered it up and took the kids to school. I went on a field trip with Buddy to the George Read house in Old New Castle. It was very nice, and I ended up staying for the rest of the day to help his teacher out. I did have to continue to take some Motrin for the discomfort, so I called Dr. Warren. She reassured me that it is normal due to the amount and tighter stitching that she did. It is not a sign of infection, yeah!

Later today, Buddy has a doctor's appointment to have his hearing rechecked. The ears were clear of infection; but his canal should "wave" when air is blown through it, and his does not, which means that fluid can still be behind the ear. There is no antibiotic that would clear it up. The doctor retested with their hearing test, and again Buddy failed. He only heard two beeps. I asked if I could try it, thinking that it didn't work. And let me tell you, you REALLY have to concentrate to hear those beeps, but it did work. We were going to hold off on any referrals to an ENT, but when he heard that we have been dealing with this for about a year, the doctor said, "Let's get him to an ENT and get a consultation for possible tubes to clear the passageway." So now we need to make an appointment with Dr. Luft. We are going to hold off on any meds, i.e., Concerta until we get the hearing taken care of. Solve one problem at a time.

We picked up Zachary, got some Mickey Ds, and headed off to Cub Scouts. Later at night, Buddy was complaining of a headache and stomachache. So we checked, and his temperature was ninety-nine degrees. I gave him some Advil, and we went off to bed.

Wednesday, January 16, 2008

HERE COMES THE GOOD NEWS! It was doctor and chemo day today, and Dad was going to take me. But we were keeping Buddy home from school because he still had a fever, so Dad stayed with him. I would be okay to go by myself because my friend Kathy was going to be there for her first treatment. And if anything happens to me, I am sure they will help me out. I got there, and Kathy was a little nervous because she just got her port placed on Monday, and they were going to access it today. I would have been nervous too. She was glad to see me, but I couldn't stay for support because they were waiting to take my blood. I had the blood taken and went back over to Kathy. She made out fine; they used some freezing spray, and she didn't feel a thing. I went to wait for the doctor, and here it comes . . . He said that since I had a reaction to Taxol later on the other night, it confirms that I am allergic to Taxol, and he wants to stop my treatment! I was not sure how I felt about the news; I knew that I should have been happy, but I was scared at the same time. What if there is still something in my body that the first two treatments didn't get, and now he is stopping it? I felt like my security blanket was being taken away from me. He reassured me and brought up the study again that showed that with the type of breast cancer that I had, Taxol didn't show any effect. But if you can remember, I had asked him in the beginning about that study, and he still wanted to do Taxol. He said that he would not feel right giving me Taxol and me having a more severe reaction this time, knowing that I really do have an allergy to it. Basically, the risk outweighs the benefit of trying it one more time. So I had to trust his judgment, and we stopped treatment. So no more chemo! As I said before, my reaction was a confusing one. You almost feel that chemo is a security, and now it is being taken away. I know that I would feel the same way on my last treatment. He wanted me to start the Tamoxifen right away, and this will be taken for five years. He went over the side effects of increased hot flashes, possible discharge, possibly no more menstrual periods; but they may come back in a year or two. I need to let him know if I have any severe leg pain because it can cause a blood clot, and I have to make sure that I get annual OB checks because it can thicken the endometrial wall, which may cause cancer. Oh great! I am scheduled to see the radiation oncologist on January 24th to discuss when I can start radiation, but I have to wait at least two weeks up to two months before I start. This is a good thing because now I have some time for the wound to heal up nicely and get re-inflated before they start radiation. After twenty-eight days of radiation, I will then get the implants placed and my port removed at the same time. They wanted to take the port out today, but Dr. Warren said that she would remove it if Dr. Biggs was okay with leaving it in for a couple of months. I just have to go and get it flushed once a month.

I went and shared my news with Kathy and the nurses, and everyone was so excited. I think that I was in shock. I hung out with Kathy anyway and kept her company. I finally left at noon and went to Dr. Strasser and set my appointment. When I left, I ran into a very dear friend of mine. I sat with her for a while and updated her since she didn't know too much about was going on with me. She was actually there with a friend of hers who was getting treatment. It was great seeing her. I then went to Dr. Warren and shared the news with her. She was very happy that the chemo was stopped so that we can get some good healing. Pray, pray for that! Finally, I called Bill and the rest of my family to fill them in on the news, and all of their reactions were the same. We almost sounded disappointed, but at the same time, we were very happy! I was on a floating cloud knowing that my "rough" days are behind me, and I was ready to move on to the next step. Later at night, we had dinner, and Buddy stayed with Joanne. He doesn't have a fever anymore, but I still wanted him to rest. I took Zachary to wrestling practice. I was still excited, nervous, and confused.

Thursday, January 17, 2008

So here we are today, and I just don't know what to do with myself. I was feeling great, still a little nervous, but it was settling in. What can I get into next—cleaning, organizing, finally getting my summer clothes away, and getting my winter clothes out. Oh, but wait, I still have to watch what I do because excessive lifting can damage the sutures that are trying to heal, and just because I didn't get chemo doesn't mean that the range of motion is back to normal. Okay, so I was getting a little ahead of myself, but anyway, I am feeling great, and I was happy with the news. But, good things do have to come to an end though; they informed me that my hair will start to grow back in about two weeks. Any other person would be happy with this news. But let me tell you, they forgot they were talking to the furry monster, and the hair on my legs was starting to grow back already. It is softer coming out, but I know that will change, and I was kind of getting used to my bald head and not having to deal with my hair. I am anxious to see what color my hair really is and how it will come out. But you know that I will keep you posted on that as well.

Well, that is it for now, and again I want to thank everyone for your generous thoughts, gifts, and offer of support during my chemo Tx's. I am sorry that all of you didn't get a chance to sit in with me, but I am sure that we can think of other ways to get together in a better atmosphere. They say that during radiation, there is a cumulative effect of tiredness, and it usually hits you on the second week. But I think I can handle being tired. If you want to visit me, then I am sure that I won't be as active. But you never know. I told Dr. Biggs that he forgot he was dealing with Superwoman here, and I will get through this the strong way. So again, I want to thank all of you for everything, and I hope that you are enjoying the updates.

Hugs to you all,
Sharon

Another reason that I continued to write my updates/journal is the responses that I got back from friends. Here is an example:

Hey Sharon! I just love your emails . . . particularly this one. You are an inspiration, you really are. I am praying for you and wish you the VERY, VERY BEST. I am so glad to hear you're done with chemo. I just wanted to say thanks again for your brave candidness with every e-mail you send. To be honest, as scary as I think it would be to have cancer, I know what to expect now. I don't want to say it would "ease" it, but I would feel more comfortable, I guess. I'm not doing a very good job of getting out what I want to say, LOL. I hope you know what I mean. You have paved the way, prepared us in a way, and I want to thank you for that. You are an amazing woman. Please keep me updated as you have been. I hope someday your boys realize how awesome of a mom they really have! GOD BLESS YOU!

Love,
Vicki R.

I will not be giving you a day-to-day account of my activities because honestly things have slowed down quite a bit. YEAH!

THINGS ARE SLOWING DOWN!

Friday, January 18 to Tuesday, January 22, 2008

There really isn't much to report. I have been continually working on getting my strength back. My energy level is getting there as well. So during this time, I am thoroughly enjoying being able to be there for my kids and NOT being so stressed out.

Wednesday, January 23, 2008

Today is Zachary's fifth birthday! He was so excited and now he thinks that he can get on the bus with Buddy and go to school. We took him to Lone Star for dinner on Monday, and the staff came out and sang Happy Birthday to him. He was a little scared at first, and then when he realized that they were singing to him, he was fine. Afterwards he leaned over to me and whispered, "Mommy, thank you for singing Happy Birthday to me!" Don't you just love it?

His school had a field trip to the DuPont Theatre, and I brought in cupcakes and then took him home early. We had wrestling practice at night, so we didn't do much else. There was no time for cancer talk on this day; this is Zachary's day.

Thursday, January 24, 2008

I had my appointment with Dr. Strasser, radiation oncologist. As we were getting ready to leave for the appointment, I looked down and noticed that my shirt was all wet. I tell you, there is never a dull moment. I went in, and lo and behold, my little wound has said hello to me. I changed my bandage, and we went on our way.

Dr. Strasser was very laid-back and has a good sense of humor, right down my alley. Anyway, he discussed with us that we cannot start radiation until I have better healing on my "open wound." He however does not want to wait any longer than the end of February. He does not feel that I am going to be fully healed AND fully expanded by that time. If the healing is complete, which he feels will be, then we will proceed with the radiation.

As far as the expansion goes, we will try to get what we can but we will have to finish after. This means that it may take longer to expand since my skin will lose some of its elasticity from the radiation. But again, remember that you are dealing with Superwoman, and I will show them. HA! He knows that it would be great if we could have everything pertaining to the reconstruction complete prior to it, but he did state that my health is more important than the cosmetics. Ya think! He did not go over any of the specifics this time, and said he wanted to see me after three weeks. He did show me how I need to have my arm during the Tx, and oh my, I need some work right there. He still feels that the twenty-eight txs are what we will do. The nurse did give me a "halter-top" type of bandage to wear over the gauze since my skin is getting irritated again from the tape. So I got to play with that at home. Meanwhile, I continued to leak and needed to be prepared wherever I go. Later today, we had our school conference with Buddy's teacher. He has gone down some in his work, but still doing well. Mrs. Phillips stated that most of her kids went down, and she thinks it was because of the holiday.

Friday, January 25, 2008

Today is Zachary's friend's birthday party with his friends, but because of the circumstances, we took him and his best friend Trey to Chuck E. Cheese. Everyone had a great time! It is so wonderful to watch your kids enjoy themselves. You don't have to have a huge party for them to have fun.

Monday, January 28, 2008

I decided to go to the gym to exercise and stretch since it is closer than going over to Newark (where my physical therapy is, but I am on hold with that right now). I have not been to the gym in so long, but it was nice to be back. While I was there, I saw a pink box with an advertisement; and where you see pink, you think of breast cancer. Anyway, it is about a girl (twenty-seven), who is undergoing breast cancer Tx. I got a contact for her, and I have since started talking with her. She is letting me know how radiation is going.

I am meeting some very nice people during all of this.

Tuesday, January 29, 2008

I have an appointment with Dr. Warren. She was very happy with my healing and said that the "drainage" is normal because she doesn't have a very tight seal on the left side. She wanted to see me back next week, and she might close it up more, which may mean no more embarrassing moments.

She also does not feel that I will be able to heal and fully expand by the end of February, but she did say that we might be able to get half of the expansion done, and then we will get the other half done at a slower pace after radiation. She does not want me to go back to physical therapy until next week, but she does want me to continue with light stretches. I have now started taking a multivitamin and a calcium tablet. I know I should have been doing that anyway, but I never stuck with it.

Thursday, January 31, 2008

This would have been my last chemo treatment! I am very happy that I am done. My Tamoxifen came in the mail today. How ironic. I will start this tomorrow.

Friday, February 1, 2008

The sun was not shining; it was raining and cold. But you know what? It was a great day! It doesn't take the weather to make me happy anymore! I took my vitamins and my Tamoxifen (the first in the next five years!). I have just emptied my medicine basket. It was nice to get rid of all of those meds. My pile is much smaller now.

On a very happy note, my brother-in-law has safely made it home from Iraq for a nice two-week visit. My sister and Dave have been waiting very long for this. They will be going to Vermont for a couple of R-and-R days, and then we can go to see him. Your continued prayers for him and the others are greatly appreciated.

Here is an update on how I am doing. I am feeling good and continue to take one day at a time. I continue to be a little disappointed that the hair is there on my legs, but it is softer than before, and I am afraid to shave. It might come back thicker like it was. No worries though, I will eventually shave. My underarm hair is starting to grow back, and it is official, I have no more eyebrows! Oh wait, I do have ONE left on the left side! I now have to pencil them in and watch that I don't wipe it off during the day. I have been wearing my glasses to take the people's attention away from the no-eyebrows and my very little eyelashes on the bottom. My head has a shadow, and the hair is like peach fuzz. I am sure there will be more grey hair than I remember, but we will wait and see. My fingers are getting better, but my toes are still pretty numb, and when it is cold and I don't have socks or slippers on, it feels worse. I am ready for that to get back to normal. I also feel very achy in my lower back. When I get up, I feel like an old woman. I continue to have my hot flashes, and the Tamoxifen may increase those. I still have not had my menstrual cycle, and who knows if or when I will get that. I won't be too disappointed if it doesn't return!

Doesn't all of this sound fun? I am so glad that none of you have had to go through this, but if you do it won't be a surprise. You now know that you can get through it. For all of you who have gone through this, I am sure it brings back some "fun" memories. The prayers and cards continue to come, and I again, thank you for those. My hubby is enjoying putting together Team Survivor for the Relay for life. Thank you to all of those who have joined the team and/or sponsored us. We should have a great time!

I continue to help others who are going through chemo. My close friend, who I met through this process, is starting to lose her hair. I am getting her through this. We laugh and have some very interesting conversations—conversations that only "we" would understand and can talk to each other about. It is very important to have someone like that.

—

133

Moving right along!

Tuesday, February 5, 2008

I had an appointment with Dr. Warren, and she, again, was happy with my healing. But she wanted to put three stitches in the left side to try and close it up more quickly. She said that it may stop the leaking. She got me numb and stitched away. I didn't really feel anything, but I knew that she was there. I need to continue with Bacitracin and bandage two times a day. It is amazing to me how skin forms. I thought that it would be right on top, and I would see it forming, but it is forming underneath the yellow granulation tissue that I have been looking at forever. Some of that has wiped off, and there you see it, fresh skin! She will see me back after one week and wanted me to wait till next week before going back to therapy.

Wednesday, February 6, 2008

I spent the day at the HGC with my friend Kathy who was on her second Tx. Well, she certainly made it "exciting." She had a reaction to Taxotere, like five minutes into the Tx. Her mom and I were there with her, and as we said, thank God her hubby wasn't there to see it. It was so ironic how it happened. She was doing really well, and the nurse had asked how she was feeling. She said that she felt a little nauseated but thought it was from Decadron. She then asked what she would be feeling, and as the nurse was telling her, she started to see spots, have trouble breathing, and her face turned bright red in color. Well, she did just that. In a matter of seconds, she said she was feeling something and that she was seeing spots. As she was trying to push her recliner back, the nurse called for Dr. Biggs and stopped the drip; and three to four other nurses came over. One was applying the oxygen. She stated that she was starting to have trouble breathing, and her face and chest turned bright red. Dr. Biggs was there very quickly, and they give her a shot of Benadryl and Decadron. Well, when they give the IV Decadron, if it is aspirated too quickly, then you can get a burning feeling in the coochie-coo area, and oh did she have that! It doesn't last long, but she did do a little dance in the chair! Everything was calming down; her breathing was becoming easier. Still she was seeing some spots, (which, she explained, weren't black like passing out, they were white like fireworks) and her color was getting back to normal. Dr. Biggs looked over at me and wanted to know what I was doing there and told me that I was bad karma! I knew that he was joking, but when he came back to check on her, he felt bad for saying that and apologized. I reassured him that I didn't take it personally! Anyway, they started the med at a slower drip (sounds familiar), and the rest of the day was a breeze for her. Now, she had the adverse reaction to the meds, and I had the true allergic reaction. Seeing what she went through, I am glad that I only had to see it and not experience it. I am glad that I was there with her, and she was a true trouper during the whole thing. Unfortunately, it will be fear of the known versus fear of the unknown at the next Tx. But I won't be going with her so she will not have any problems! Love you, Kathy! Also, while I was there, I ran into another friend of mine who was with a friend of hers. Her friend, whom I met when she was going through radiation, was not doing so well. She had fallen and was waiting to get her strength to do the chemo. My prayers are with her and her family. We ended the day by going to PureBread Deli for a nice lunch; their lobster bisque soup is AWESOME!

Saturday, February 9, 2008

We had a wrestling tournament for Buddy, but he suddenly got "sick" while we were there. He warmed up and then came and told me that his belly hurt, crying and all. I was unsure if he was telling the truth, considering that the stomach virus was going around and there were two other boys who didn't make it that day. Bill kept telling me that he was fine and that he would have to get sick on the mat before he took him out. We had him wrestle his first match, and then we forfeited the next, which Bill hated to do. We changed and headed home. When we got in the car, he asked if he could have a donut! Oh my gosh, he just played me! We made him lie in bed all day, and later, he admitted that he was not sick and that it was more nerves than anything. Hey, you live and learn. My motherly instinct was to take care of him, and Bill's fatherly instinct told him, "Been there, done that." This was new for me and Buddy too! He apologized to Bill, and we moved on.

Sunday, February 10, 2008

We go to Connections Church in Middletown for Scout Sunday. It is a very different church, very contemporary, hard to get used to, but I understood the message. Went to my parents for lunch and then Joanne and I went to Target with the kids. While I was there, my feet really felt weird. This numb feeling is so hard to get used to, but on the bright side, I haven't had any leaking incidents.

Monday, February 11, 2008

My appointment with Dr. Strasser was very short. He came in and looked at the wound and said, "We still need more healing," and "I will see you back in two weeks." The nurse, Karen, explained to me what will probably go on at the next visit. I will need to get a CAT scan and get measured for my "tattooing." It will take about one and a half hours. We will keep our fingers crossed.

Tuesday, February 12, 2008

I have an appointment with Dr. Warren at 7:45 a.m. She was again happy with the healing. She removed some of the old sutures. I explained to her that the leaking stopped on the left side, but it went over to the right side! She explained to me that the corners are the hardest for healing, and she debated putting another stitch in. She didn't want to disturb any of the new skin but decided to put in one stitch anyway. She gave me the okay to go back to therapy, which was good because I had an appointment right after. She will see me back in one week.

My therapy went well, and Lisa got updated on what has been happening. She could tell I was a little tighter than when I left, but we will get to work on it.

Wednesday, February 13, 2008

I get a call from school that Buddy came to the nurse's office in the morning, went back to class, and after lunch, he fell asleep in class. I picked him up, and he was down the rest of the day and night with a one-hundred-one-degree fever. Last week, Zachary had a slight fever, and Joanne and I noticed that his cheeks were so red. Well, she looked it up, and we thought he had "slap-cheek virus." You know, Fifth's disease. Well, once the cheeks turn red, they are not contagious any longer. Lo and behold, Buddy gets it. This was another "Mother of the Year" moment.

Thursday, February 14, 2008

Happy Valentine's Day! I woke up, and I couldn't get out of bed. I was so achy, and I thought I had a fever! Bill was on day work, and I didn't have the energy to take Zachary to school. So we lay in my bed—all three of us—all day. Buddy was starting to feel better. Zachary was in his glory because he was able to play the PSP all day, and Buddy was on the laptop. I felt like I was going through chemo all over again! It's funny though, when I was going through chemo, I would do anything to try and get up and do something. I noticed that when I was sick, I didn't want to get up for nothing, and I did just that. The kids were great and let me sleep somewhat.

We had a very dear friend from the firehouse pass away today. Vinnie Mac, as we called him, had gone in for a hernia operation; but when they opened him up, they found he had advance stages of pancreatic cancer. He did not make it long after that, so our prayers are with him. He is going to be a big loss to the firehouse and to Buddy. He loved Vinnie Mac!

Friday, February 15, 2008

It was twenty-four hours later, and I was good to go. Buddy was supposed to have his appointment with Dr. Luft. But they wanted him non-congested before checking him out, so we cancelled it. Dr. Luft wouldn't see him until March 26! Brenda and Dave came over and visited for a little while. Dave is enjoying his stay here and is not looking forward to going back to Iraq. I showed Brenda and Joanne this little "bubble," and it was giving me the urge to pop it, but I won't. I am unsure of what it is and can't wait to see Warren.

I did a Longaberger® show at my friend Amy's, and we had a blast. I was very surprised with what they did for me. I was given a Willow Tree, Angel of Miracles. She said that she has been inspired by me. She also gave me a foot bath, did some reflexology, and something else, but I don't know what it was called. It was great, nothing that I expected in doing a home show.

Saturday, February 16, 2008

I went to therapy in the morning, and when the doctor was done, she noticed that I was quite stuffy, so she did some sinus relief on me. I am getting all kinds of special treatment these days. I instantly am feeling relief.

—

Sunday, February 17, 2008

We went to a wrestling tournament in New Jersey. Buddy got third, and Zachary got a participation trophy. There were no upset stomachs this time! Brenda had a rough day because Dave left for another three to four months, but they had a great time while he was here. Please pray for his safe return!

Monday, February 18, 2008

Buddy had an appointment with Kym, the psychologist, and she felt that he was doing well. He did mention to her about Vinnie Mac and she said he may need to talk about it. She was okay to see him in two months, unless he needs to talk about something when I am going through the radiation. He has also been participating in a lunch bunch at school, which is a group of kids who have family members going through rough times. They get together every other week, discuss any concerns, and play games. I think all of this is helping him deal with my cancer.

Tuesday, February 19, 2008

I had a therapy appointment, and it was a really good one. I felt really loose on my trap muscle, and my range is getting better.

Wednesday, February 20, 2008

I saw Dr. Warren, and she continued to be happy with the healing and the suturing on the left side coming together. The bubble on the right side that I saw was some thin skin. She popped it, drains it some, and then tried to suture it. But the new skin was not strong enough and kept tearing, so she needed to suture it at a different angle, and oh did I feel that. I am starting to get a little bit of feeling, and it is bittersweet. She said that I shouldn't feel any more discomfort than what I am feeling now and that she will see me back in a week. When I left, I got the feeling that I didn't want to move because it was pulling and felt tight. I didn't want the suture to rip or break even though she reassured me that I will be okay. I kept getting a sharp pain, and I took a couple of Motrin. I went to bed on the early side and rested.

Thursday, February 21, 2008

I woke up, and I was a little sore and nervous to go to therapy, but I knew that I had to go. When I got there, the doctor started stretching me and could tell that I was nervous. She and I figured out that where I was feeling the tightness was far from where the suture was. My tightness was actually in my pectoral muscle, so I got a little more relaxed. She worked on my chording that was still going on. She couldn't believe that I just couldn't catch a break, but we knew that it was all good.

Friday, February 22, 2008

Today, school was closed due to snow. I was not feeling as tight or as much discomfort, but I was still being protective. No doctor's visits today. Yeah!

Now, for my body-appearance update. I have shaved my legs once, and either the razor was dull or I am growing hair like an animal because it is long again! The underarms have been shaved, and that was okay. The eyebrows, believe it or not, are starting to come back out already! They are fuzzy and salt-and-pepper-looking. My eyelashes are also growing nicely. While talking to my mom yesterday, she was asking how the hair growth was coming, and I went into the bathroom and was looking at myself in the mirror. I was not sure that was a good idea because, oh my gosh, I looked like I have a beard. I was so fuzzy. Was I this bad before? Don't tell me. Anyway, I will deal with this as it comes. My hair on my head is growing back quickly, very salt-and-pepper-looking and very soft. The kids are excited to see this and like to touch it. It will be interesting to see how it will grow back. My nails keep breaking very low, and I just accept that it is the chemo getting out of my body and that they will be the way they were soon. Other than that, all is good. I continue to take one day at a time and enjoy that I am feeling good and have energy. When I talk to you again, I will have had my appointment with Strasser and may have a better idea about when I will start radiation. Until then, go and enjoy the snow, be safe, and hug someone you love.

COUPLE OF SAD DAYS.

Saturday, February 23, 2008

B ill and I went to our friend Vinnie's funeral. It was very touching, and
we all will miss him very much. He was a good man as Buddy said.
I am a little concerned with my site as the "bubble" is starting to reappear!
It looks like a whitish bubble, and I just want to push on it to get the fluid
out, but I don't. Man why can't this thing just heal already! I continued to
leak, and I changed the dressing as usual. The discomfort has gone away, but
my chording is getting painful. STRETCH, STRETCH, STRETCH!

Monday, February 25, 2008

I saw Dr. Strasser (radiation oncologist), and it was another
less-than-two-minute visit. I told him that my Superwoman powers are
failing me! He looked at the site and said, "Okay, we are going to give it
another two weeks." I asked him if he was okay with that, and he said that
one can't rush healing. He definitely would like to have started sooner, but
we can't with it being open like that. He also would like to have all of the
stitches out prior to starting. I scheduled for Friday, March 7, in hopes
that things will look better. I called and let everyone know, as I usually
do, and the same questions came about. Do you think this is normal? Is
it because of the chemo that you are taking so long to heal? How are you
feeling? Well, of course I would say it is not "normal," you ultimately would
like to have no reaction to the dye and go straight to healing like I did on
the right side. Part of it is due to the chemo for the length of time that
it is taking it to heal, but Warren said the last time that the corner is the
toughest place to heal. Yes, I am feeling okay, but I am ready to get started
with the next phase.

Tuesday, February 26, 2008

I had therapy in the morning, and I was there for about one and a half hours. I was explaining what was going on, and Lisa looked at the site to make sure that she was not stretching it too much. She noticed the leaking and the "bubble." Lisa looked at me and said, "You just can't get a break, can you?" Hey, what are you going to do, things could be a lot worse. I just go with the flow. The stretching is helping with the chording, and she was just concerned that I do not get lymphodema! Can you imagine if I had to add that to my list of "problems"? I continued with the rest of my program, and she reminded me to stretch three times a day.

Wednesday, February 27, 2008

I was taking Zachary to school, and Joanne called me and told me some very upsetting news. You know my inspiration during this whole ordeal has been Wendi Fox Pedicone. She has been so strong in her battle with cancer. But it finally came to an end. My brother-in-law saw the obituary in the paper and called to tell us. Joanne and I were in silence, not knowing what to say. Joanne said that her last updates have not been that positive and that they didn't sound good. I went to Wawa after I dropped off Zachary and got a paper; I read it and just couldn't believe that she was gone. She was such a fighter. I came home, started on the computer, went to her websiteFoxpress. com—and looked and read her last two updates. As I was reading the updates, I became so upset and just broke down in tears. I think it was just a reality check. I was thinking that that could be me. She fought her breast cancer, but then had a recurrence that went to the liver and other areas. She just couldn't beat it this time. She has four kids—one is almost as young as my boys—and a very loving husband who has been so supportive with her whole process. She never gave up, and it hurt to know that she didn't fight it. But that will give me even more courage and strength to fight and beat this dreaded disease. This is for her! So in your prayers, please add her family to that list, and just remember, life is short, and you never know what you will be dealt with. You need to enjoy life, family, work, and to be alive. Don't take things for granted, and if there is something that you keep thinking of doing, and you just haven't done it, well, I guess now is the time! I hug all of you right now and thank you for being a part of my life! Okay, I need to move on; the eyes are filling up.

My girlfriend Merith came over and brought me some lunch (and dinner), and I had to explain to her why my eyes were all red. We had a

---

great three hours that we just sat and caught up about things. She is about to have surgery next Wednesday to correct her eye from the thyroid cancer, but like me, she goes with the flow and tries to find any reason to laugh and have a good time (with her and me, that is not hard to do). Friends are the best!

Later that night, I went to the firehouse to a Ladies' Auxiliary function, and my mom has joined with a friend of hers, Pat. I was happy to see that my mom has joined so she could have something to do and to know that this is something that we will be able to do together. Is there something that you can do with your mom or dad? Take the time to do it; it means so much to you and to them!

Thursday, February 28, 2008

I had an early appointment with Dr. Warren. She looked at the site and explained to me what was going on. The "bubble," that is there is granulation tissue, but there is NO skin underneath that, and my expander is exposed! I felt like I was having a déjàvu! What she was having a problem doing was suturing to strong tissue. The new tissue that has formed has not been strong enough to hold the skin together, and that is why the bubble keeps forming. I asked her if we needed to deflate more to create more skin to pull from, but she said, "No, there is enough skin, I just need to find the right angle to get it to stay."

We are trying so hard to stay away from any grafting, and she is seeing continual healing. That is why she is not giving up going this route. So she numbed me, and oh, I felt that. She was quiet for a minute or two, and then she got to work. She put in three to four new stitches in hopes that these would work. She advised me not to do any stretching for the next couple of days to give this a chance to stay together. Here we go, one step forward and two steps back. I was just starting to get some relief on the chording, and now I can't stretch. Oh well, what are you going to do?" I did ask her if, even though it's not going to happen, the bubble reappears, should I come in sooner than a week to get it closed again? She said that if it is leaking, no problem, but if the "bubble" appears again, then I should come in sooner. Otherwise, she will see me next week.

I left her office and informed my family about what was going on. I am planning on going to square one again and do hardly anything—no vacuuming, lifting clothes baskets, etc, etc. I will do whatever it takes to get this closed.

I got home and basically sat in front of the computer all day. That doesn't require much lifting, just remembering to sit up straight. At about two thirty in the afternoon, the numbness was starting to wear off. I was feeling some discomfort. I took some Motrin in hopes that it would relieve it. I took it easy the rest of the night. Bill took care of dinner, and the kids and I played on Webkinz. We called it a night and tried to get a comfortable sleep.

Friday, February 29, 2008

The night was a little rough; I was trying not to move too much as I have gotten in the habit of stretching my arm out for the chording. Needless to say, I was up quite a bit. When I changed the bandage today, all continued to look good. No sign of the "bubble"! I went to Zachary's school, did a dental presentation, came home, had lunch, and finished this update. I was feeling a little rundown, so I thought that I would go lie down until the Budman gets home. My sisters and I are going to New York tomorrow on a bus trip, so you know that I need to get prepared. My mom was supposed to go, but she was insisting that I go since I am not undergoing treatment right now. We will pray for nice weather, and I will make sure that I am fully prepared for any leakage. Won't that just be a situation! Have a great day!

Oh yeah, the personal appearance. The hair continues to grow, can't see any chemo curl yet, but it is so soft. My eyebrows are getting darker as they come back. The eyelashes are coming back quick. Of course, the leg and "middle" area is in full swing! I realized that I did lose some arm hair, but since I was so hairy on my arms, it wasn't as noticeable, but it did thin out. I thank those of you who reassured me that I wasn't that hairy on my face prior to chemo, but I am not sure if I believe you, LOL. My nails are getting stronger, yeah. My back continues to give me problems when I get up from sitting; and my big toe is still numb but definitely is getting better! I have been faithfully taking my Tamoxifen, multivitamin, and calcium tablet daily. I think that is my body in a nutshell. I hope you get the visual! I will continue to keep you posted, and as I said, don't put off till tomorrow what you can or plan on doing today! Make sure you hug someone today and share your feelings with the one whom you love. You never know what life will bring you.

Spring will soon be here!

Saturday, March 1, 2008

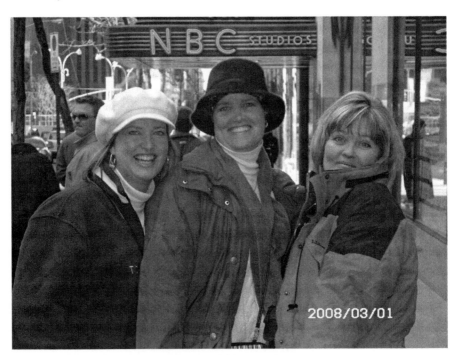

A day in New York City with my sisters

My sisters, some friends, and I went on a bus trip to New York. The day was beautiful! We toured NBC studios, went to St. Patrick's Cathedral (I think that is the name, it is beautiful!), saw Hairspray, ate at ESPN zone, and left to come home. The show was awesome. Norm from

Cheers was the Mom. He was very funny, but I just knew that he was going to have a heart attack right on stage because of his weight. I know that some of it was fluff, but WOW! Anyway, the seats were great. We were four rows back. Thank you, Little Brenda, I had a great time! I didn't have any catastrophes with leakage. In fact, Brenda went into the bathroom with me at the theater, and we just added more bandage instead of exposing the area. You know, with all the germs, we decided to play it safe. The weather wasn't that cold so my feet did pretty good. My sister-in-law watched the boys, and they went to Xbos and had a great time. It was a great time spent with my sisters.

Sunday, March 2, 2008

Buddy had his Pinewood Derby for Cub Scouts. We got fourth place each time he raced, but we had a good time. We will work more on it next year!

Everything is still closed, and we are hoping it stays that way! It was a pretty laid-back day after that.

Tuesday, March 4, 2008

I had therapy in the morning, and we saw a little opening, Oh crap! Lisa was careful with the stretching and reassured me that everything is going to be okay. Her sister was recently diagnosed with breast cancer and had her surgery on Friday! When is it going to stop!

I went to get my oil changed in the hoopty (Bill's neon car that he drives to work, great on gas!). Then I went to Costco to rotate the tires and get some necessities. Can't you just go crazy in there? (Costco, that is.)

Later that night, we dropped the boys off at our friends' house for Cub Scouts, and we went to the kickoff meeting for the relay for life. It sounds like we are going to have a great time at relay. They have activities all throughout the day and night. I have a feeling it will be a little emotional but a really fun time. We are looking forward to it. Bill and I are working on putting together a Beef-and-Beer to raise money for ACS, but that is still in the making. Thank you to all of you who have donated and/or are a part of our team. I hope to make this an annual event.

Wednesday, March 5, 2008

Oh phooey! Guess what? My area has opened again! I dropped the boys off to school and headed over to Dr. Warren's. When I got there, I found out she would be in surgery all day. But they gave me an appointment for tomorrow at 1:30 p.m. I am trying not to blame myself, but here it goes. Maybe I was good the first couple of days, but then I started to do too much. Maybe I should have, could have, didn't . . . Oh stop! It is open now, and there is nothing you can do about it now!

Later tonight was Wendi's memorial. We have not seen it advertised anywhere, but my therapist found out where and when it would be held. Joanne, Kathy, and I planned on attending. It was from six to nine in the evening at the Hockessin fire hall. We were not sure what to expect, but were glad we are able to go. My friend Kathy was having a down day and was unsure if she should go tonight. She has one more chemo treatment to go, and this was her time when was feeling yucky. I agreed with her that she was better off not going due to the amount of people that are going to be there, and since her counts are probably down, she doesn't want to end up in the hospital again.

Joanne and I got there, and the parking lot was full and very messy, to say the least (they are doing some construction on it, and it was very muddy!). I was feeling a little uncomfortable since I knew we wouldn't know anyone and because I have chosen to wear my scarf versus my wig. We went in, and there was a picture of her and her family, a donation box for Danny's college fund, and her book to take for a donation that you give. There were tables set up, and tons of people were there, enjoying each other's company. There were many pictures of her and her family everywhere. While we were looking around, I ran into some of my patients, and they were shocked because they were unaware of my diagnosis. They also were telling me that they are not letting anyone touch their teeth until I return to work. It is great to feel wanted, but I reassured them that it will be okay and told them to keep up with their dental health. What a hygienist! Anyway, a friend of the family spoke for a little, and then there was a slide presentation, and it was great. I thought, *Oh no, this is going to be a tearjerker. Get the tissues ready.* But you know what, it wasn't. It was just what Wendi wanted. There were no flowers there, and it was all about celebrating her life and the happy times that she had. There weren't any of her times during treatment or illness but happy times with her family and friends. Her husband and two of the daughters said a few words, and then it was back to socializing. I went up to Dan and thanked him for sharing Wendi with all of us, and I learned that he is just as positive as Wendi was.

While I was talking to Wendi's neighbor, Cammi, who is also a patient of mine, a girl came up to me and just wanted to thank me for wearing my scarf instead of my wig. She went on to say that she is a survivor and was glad to see that I had that on. We spoke a while, and this funny question came up again that we, newly "survivors" don't know how to answer. That question again is, "How long have you been a survivor?" We both wondered, *Is it since you are first diagnosed*, which is what Joanne had said, but "we" don't really feel that way when you are still going through treatment. It will be an easier question to answer five years from now. But wait, when is my one year anniversary? I think for me, it will be after radiation or my first checkup stating that all is still fine. Don't worry, you know that I will keep you posted. Anyway, after I was finished speaking with her, another lady came up to introduce herself. She was Wendi's cousin. She just wanted to wish me luck. She is a cancer survivor as well and was glad to see that I could make it. After that, we signed the guest book and headed for home. All in all, it was a very nice memorial, and I am very glad that I was able to attend.

On the way home, Joanne and I were talking, and I had told her that since Wendi's passing, it has opened up my eyes even more on my life. I am in a similar position as surviving breast cancer, but I am not out of the woods yet. I know no one wants to hear this, but two years from now, I could be affected again. You never know. I am not going to dwell on that thought, but I am going to make some changes in my life that I never realized needed to be done until now. Our society gets into our routines, and then we forget what is really important—being happy! Forget being stressed out and don't sweat the small stuff. Okay, my psychology session is over, I will get on with my update.

Thursday, March 6, 2008

I had my appointment with Dr. Warren, and I couldn't wait. The area looked bigger than before. It was finally one thirty in the afternoon, and she looked at the site and said, "Okay, were done playing now!" She told me that I am not going to like her news, but she is going to have to deflate me more. Hey, at this point, do what you have to do. So, she got me numb, feeling was coming back, took out sixty to ninety more CC's, and then stitched the heck out of me with the stronger tissue. She did give me a better explanation of what has happened. I asked that when the blue dye is ever used on me, do I need to inform them that I am allergic to it? She explained to me that no, the dye (methyl blue) is used for breast cancer patients to detect the node involvement. It is a dye that will kill the skin if it touches it, which is what happened to me. They are able to use it for breast cancer patients because it is injected deep in the tissue, and it will excrete through the lymphatic system. But it depends on how much is used, how much is diluted, and if the blood vessels attach to it. Well, in my case, the lovely dye came up to the skin and killed my lovely tissue. So not only did I have the slow healing from chemo, I had to grow back new skin! Lucky me. This is how I understood it, anyway. She wanted to see me back early next week to make sure there is no more opening.

As my numbness was wearing off, I began to feel some discomfort. I took some Motrin, and Bill and I went to get our taxes done. On the way home, I informed him that I was going to go right to bed when I get home since I am hurting. Funny thing is that I was not hurting where the stitches are; I was hurting where the muscle/tissue was being pulled tight. I got on my PJs and figured that since the Motrin didn't take it away and I am not going to be driving anywhere, I should just go ahead and take a Percocet. Now the pain wasn't excruciating, but it was constant. And after getting my taxes done, which I got so nervous about, it was nice to not worry about anything and relax before, I took Percocet before I was taking it prior to any pain, so I guessed it worked. This time, when I took it, I had pain prior to taking it. Hey, it really works. My pain was gone, and I was very relaxed! I had a pretty good night. Bill, on the other hand, had to deal with the kids, and like I said, I didn't worry about anything. Bill was asking for one by the end of the night!

Friday, March 7, 2008

I had a good night, but I am feeling really tired today. I left Zachary home. Joanne came over to check on me. Jaylyn and Zachary played nicely while Joanne and I were catnapping. She seems to always blame me for not getting anything done around her house! Hey remember, don't sweat the small stuff, it will be there later on! The pain was still there, but the relaxing did help. I didn't take any more meds and just hung low. Bill was so faithful in calling to check up on me and make sure I am okay. I love you, Bill!

Weekend was nice, busy with baseball meetings and practices for the boys. Good news, everything is still closed. I continue to leak but I will take that.

Monday, March 10, 2008

I had an appointment with Warren, and it was pretty boring! We like boring. She was happy with the way it looks and wanted to see me back on Thursday since she will be away all of next week. Fine with me, see ya!

Tuesday, March 11, 2008

I have no doctor's visits today. I was watching Jaylyn. Zachary was in preschool, and Buddy and Jessica have DSTP testing this week. Hope all goes well.

Wednesday, March 12, 2008

Can you believe it, no doctor's visits again today! Buddy has had a couple of bad days at school with calling out, making noises, and talking back to the teacher. She had called yesterday to inform me and talk to him, and then I got another phone call today asking if I would like to talk to him again or come in. I decided to go in and see what's going on. I was curious if he is worrying about me. But at the same time, he was doing testing. The room looked different, his schedule was all messed-up, and there was daylight savings time. When I went in to observe, I noticed that many of the kids were acting out, so I have made an appointment for Buddy to see Kym. But I think a lot of it has to do with all the changes. At least I hope so.

Thursday, March 13, 2008

I saw Warren today at 8:15 a.m., and she was very pleased with the way the suture looked. She will see me back in a week and a couple days. She told me to tell Strasser that she wants to leave the stitches in during radiation for stability and more healing but that nothing is open. Hopefully, tomorrow will be my day to get my tattooing, CATSCAN, and molding. And then I will start radiation the next week!

Okay, that is it for now. I know, Auxi, I get long-winded, but this is like my diary of things that have gone on in my life, and I want to remember them this way since my mind seems to forget these days. So, as I always say to you, enjoy your life, your family and your friends; and always remind yourself, DON'T SWEAT THE SMALL STUFF!

—

INTERESTING HAPPENINGS!

Friday, March 14, 2008

I had my appointment with Strasser at 1:00 p.m. Bill was off and was able to go with me. Yeah! I know that he was glad also since he has not been able to go with me the last couple of times. Dr. Strasser came in and looked at the site and was confused as to what we should do. He knew that it is healing but not completely yet, and he knew that we are past the time frame of what they like to wait for radiation after chemo. He said he is going to go get another doctor to get his opinion. He then came in and did a "photo shoot" of my breast. Watch out, Playboy! He ended up deciding on his own that we are going to go ahead with the CAT scan and tattooing. The process is going to take about forty-five minutes. Bill went to run an errand, and I went to get the CAT scan, which was right in the same office. Finally, the nurses got a face to my name since I have had to cancel so many times in the past for not being ready.

The nurse was positioning me and adjusting my arm. It's a little tight for me, but she had me resting on a "bean bag" pillow so it was bearable. The next thing I knew she was suctioning all of the air out of the pillow to create a mold where I would be laying once the treatments begin. The pillow ended up being so hard. How easy, one step done. She then lined me up and got ready for my tattoos. This was such a big day for me, Playboy and tattoos! I am such a rebel! I asked if I am aloud to pick my design and color. She responded that I can't pick my design. She only does dots, and I can pick from black, black, or black as my color. So I went for black.

My tattooing was done, one on each side and one in the middle of my stomach. These tattoos are to make sure that I am in a straight line on the table for treatment. Then I got ready for the CAT scan, no problems with that. They had a beautiful scenery picture on the light on the ceiling. When it was done, she asked me what time I would like to have for my treatments. I asked for 9:30 a.m., and the closest they could get me was 9:45 p.m. I took it. I got dressed and went back to Karen, a registered nurse. She told me not to use deodorant with aluminum and recommended that I use the Adidas deodorant. Also, she told me to use mild soap such as Ivory and Dove and non-scented lotion such as Eucerin. My start date is going to be on March 28, 2008, and that will be a trial run. I asked if I can see the radiation rooms, and she took me to the Vault. What a name for it. On the way there, she explained what the routine will be—check in, get changed, and sit to be called. I will be in the same vault for all treatments. Once I am finished with all of my treatments, there is a bell that I get to ring to signify that I am done! The rooms are huge. The door thickness is from my fingertips to past my elbow! There is another nice scenery on the ceiling, and she says they will have the music on for relaxation. I feel like I am at the spa! Behind the wall are all of the molds. They each have their own cubby. I am sorry that Bill missed this part, but I will get him to see it next time. My appointment was done, and now I just wait for the twenty-eighth.

Saturday, March 15, 2008

Pretty busy day! We got up in the morning for the Easter Egg Hunt at Delaware River Bay at ten. It was very windy and cold, but the kids had a great time. Joanne took Zachary, and I left for baseball practice for Buddy, which was at eleven in the morning. Practice was over at one in the afternoon, and then Buddy and I headed to set up for the Blue/Gold dinner for Cub Scouts. We got that done and then went home to get ready for the dinner. Bill surprised us by getting off of work early and being able to go. It was a nice evening, and Buddy got his Wolf badge. My mom was able to go, and that was also nice that she was able to make it. We questioned whether or not we think Buddy will continue when he gets to Boy Scouts.

Sunday, March 16, 2008

The kids and I went to Cornerstone Presbyterian Church to see if we like it, and everyone was very nice and welcoming. I felt very guilty going to another church since my church has been very supportive during my diagnosis. My reasoning to look at a different church is due to the Sunday school for the kids. I want them to learn and feel the importance of the church, and we don't really have that opportunity at my present church. My girlfriend Merith helped me to feel a little better about this. After church, we went to my parents for lunch and a quick visit, headed home, and just enjoyed the day.

Monday, March 17, 2008

I got out of the shower, checked out the area, and to no surprise, there was a teeny tiny area that looked to be opening! I took Zachary to school and headed right over to Dr. Warren's to have nurse look at it since she is away for the week. Christine looked at it, and when she wiped it off, the floodgates opened again. She put some gauze on it and said she would call the doctor on call to suture it closed or at least take a look. The doctor on call was a doctor in Wilmington. I got in my car and headed in that direction of his office. I figured that I can visit Joanne until my appointment. They called and asked if I could be there by 1:45 p.m. I went to Joanne's work, and she was surprised but scared to death when I told her that I need to go to another doctor's appointment. She was thinking of the worse since I had my CAT scan on Friday! I calmed her down, and we were able to have lunch together.

I headed over to the on-call doctor, but I was feeling a little nervous to see this doctor. I hear he does not have the best bedside manner, and you know how comfortable I am with Warren. As I was sitting in the reception area, there was a young family with their newborn, and in walked a mother and her daughter in her white silk pants, thong, and big sunglasses. Anyway, they started having this conversation about how painful and tight they were feeling and if it was normal. As they were comparing notes—the "new" mother and the other mother—I heard the "model wannabe" say that she is currently getting face abrasion (or something like that). Then she said, "All I know is that when I turn twenty-five, I am getting *these* bigger. Blah, blah, blah." I am not saying that no one should ever get bigger breasts, but at that particular time, I was not feeling like hearing that kind of a conversation. Enough of that. The nurse took me back, and the doctor came in—older, gray-haired man (even more gray hair than mine). He took off the bandage, and I was still leaking.

"Okay, let me lay you back."

Once he laid me back, he started pushing and squeezing my "breast." One side of me was saying, "Ouch, you're hurting me. What are you doing?" The other side of me was saying, "Okay, maybe this is what it needed to stop the leaking. But it still is uncomfortable." I explained to him what has happened and asked him if he has ever seen this. He said, "It's been a long time, I don't do this anymore."

WHAT! Oh great, now I was feeling really comfortable. He didn't see any infection but wanted to take a culture on it. He got the swab out, stuck it in there, and said, "If anything comes up, we will call you in a couple of days." He was so gentle, NOT! As he was examining, he said to me that if I was his patient, he would just take out the expander. He asked me where my port was to fill the expander, and I explained how Warren uses this magnetic device. "Oh, well, I don't even have one of those. We'll have to get it from her office." What he decided to do was try to calculate how much saline I had put in and how much she had taken out, and see if he can remove any more. He will call me once he gets the information. Once I was out the door, my floodgates opened up; but this time, it was from my eyes. I know that I am not a failure, but that word kept coming into my mind. After all of this time and with such a small area, and I had to lose the expander! I sat in the parking lot and tried to calm down, thinking of whom to call. I didn't want to call Bill or Joanne in this state because it will upset them that they couldn't be there with me. I'll call them later. I called my "breast" friend Kathy, no answer. I didn't leave a message because she won't be able to understand what I would be saying. *Okay, start driving home; it is a quarter past two in the afternoon.* My tears continued to flow but not so much that I couldn't see. I headed over to pick up Zach, but I knew that he was still sleeping, so I went to the library parking lot near his school and just sat in my car and had some time to myself. I gathered my thoughts. One side said, *Call Joanne and ask her to pick up Zach so that you can just get in bed.* The other side said, *No, if you go home, you will just lie there and get depressed. Take some time regain your thoughts and pick up Zach.* Well, this side won. I regained my thoughts so much that I even fell asleep. I felt much better when I woke up. I picked up Zach and headed home. Once Joanne got home, she took all the kids down to her house, and I made some more phone calls. The doctor's office called me and wanted me to come in tomorrow at 1:45 p.m. I was not feeling too comfortable about this man due to his bedside manner, and when I talked to a coworker who asked me if I could cancel the appointment once she heard who it was but, I told them I would be there. Brenda informed me that what he meant by "I don't do this anymore" is that he doesn't do reconstruction after a mastectomy and that he only does cosmetic surgery. Feel a little better now? Not really.

Later that night, Bill asked me what time the appointment will be and where his office is located. I thought, *He is going to try and be there for my appointment tomorrow.* We talked a good bit prior to falling asleep after a long day!

Tuesday, March 18, 2008

Kids were in school, and Bill called to tell me that he would meet me at my appointment! He was going to take leftover vacation hours to be there for me. I was worried but kept myself busy. Of course, my sisters were telling me to take Xanax before I go.

"No, I am more nervous on what I am going to feel."

"Then take a Percocet."

Oh yeah, that will be good. I will fall asleep on the table while the doctor is working on me.

"No, I will be fine. I don't need any meds."

The appointment time came, and Bill met me there. When we went back, I asked him how long it has been since he has done it, and he said about four years. He laid me back flat (normally, I am not back that much). He was using the magnetic device that the nurse from Warren's office brought over. A process that takes one minute to do with one little dot took about three minutes. I had all kinds of pen marks on me. Poor guy, you CAN tell it has been a while. He got me numb and stuck me. He tried to aspirate, but nothing was coming out. He pushed on the expander/breast and said, "This has to be the port. I can feel the bottom of the expander," as he was moving the syringe up and down. HELLO, don't pop a hole in it dude, that is all I need. (That was in my head, of course.) He tried to aspirate again but still nothing. He pulled it out and said, "Okay I can't get anything. It is against my better judgment to resuture you, so until Warren gets back, keep this dry. If it starts to get red or painful, then call me or Saunders (Warren's partner). We will be in the office on Friday. I am not going to take out your expander, because you are not my patient, and it will not hurt to leave it in until Warren is back."

I got dressed and they gave me some dressings and the magnetic device. Bill and I were on our way. Okay, I guess that wasn't too bad. I am going to have to start facing the fact that I am going to lose my expander. This means that once radiation is done, we will have to start all over. There is never a dull moment with me. I am definitely back to myself and joking to cope (remember my saying). It will all be fine.

I called and cancelled my therapy appointment and let them know that I will call back when all of this gets straightened out.

Buddy has had some really good days at school, so I figured that I would cancel his appointment with Kym, and we will just see her on the thirty-first. My office called and cancelled my appointment with Dr. Hazuda as he was having some back problems. I rescheduled for April 2 to talk about my return. It was another busy day.

Wednesday, March 19, 2008

I went to hang out with Kathy during her last long chemo Tx. She had no reaction this time. YEAH! While I was there, I was talking with another breast cancer patient who is now stage four. But you could never tell it. She is motivated and energetic, and one stylish lady. It was very nice talking with her, and we exchanged e-mails. Another new friend.

Kathy was teasing me, saying that they should hire me to just go around and be the social butterfly for the patients. Hey, not a bad idea!

I didn't stay the whole time. I went to square away my bills. By the way, it is so ridiculous what they charge. The initial oncology doctor charged me (my insurance) $350 for the initial consultation, where he examined me for about ten minutes. Once I was an established patient, the charge was $170. He spent a longer visit with me then. I know you are paying for the time they spend to go over our records, whatever! I still think it is ridiculous what things cost. On my way to my radiologist, I ran into a friend whose mother has brain cancer. It was their first visit to discuss some treatment, so it was a little tense. I, of course, with my silliness tried to bring a smile to their faces. I gave her mom a hug and gave her my support.

I went back to fill Karen in on what is going on and that my start date for radiation may be changed again! Karen told me to call her after I see Warren next week, and we will take it from there. I know that they are ready to go as I am too, but they have great office/social skills. They always have smiles on in that office.

I was finally finished with my errands and could head on home. It was another good day for Buddy in school. (He knows spring break is coming. Just kidding.)

Thursday, March 20, 2008

Dropped Buddy off at school. Zachary was with Joanne while I headed down to the sub sale at the firehouse. Mom was the first one to attend. She is really enjoying the Auxiliary!

Joanne dropped Jaylyn off later on and took Zach to school as she had a therapy appointment. When I got home, I definitely took a shower. The sub smell is stinky and stays on you even after the shower.

No school tomorrow and we are meeting the Cub Scouts at the bowling alley. Don't worry, I have already put the word out that I am not able to lift any of the balls nor will I be bowling. All of the parents were so helpful and had their eye on me. We had a great night, and some of us stayed till almost ten in the evening.

Friday, March 21, 2008

Not too much went on. Not too much motivation today. The kids were here, and I was just veging out to the point that I closed my eyes for a little on the couch. Joanne was doing some Easter shopping for me. Buddy has baseball practice tonight and it was cold. I sat in my car while Buddy practiced and Zachary was playing with a friend. As the night went on, I was feeling that my head was starting to hurt, and congestion was settling in along with a slight sore throat. Bill came to the rescue. He stopped by after work to see Buddy. He told me that he would go get them something to eat and that I needed to go home, get on my jammies and get in bed. So I did just that! When the boys got home, Buddy saw me in bed and wanted to know if could lie in bed with me. Then Zachary came back and forth. They were not loud, I don't mind; but Bill got a little upset. He told me that Buddy could sleep in with me, and he would go out on the couch. I could tell he was upset, and I later talked with him and found out that the reason he was upset was he worked all day and was looking forward to a night with the boys and watching TV. And when they would rather be with me back in the bedroom, that hurt his feelings. He wasn't feeling too loved at that moment. It is hard. I know that the boys don't really say too much, but when Mommy is not feeling well, they know it and want to comfort me during that time. It is not that they don't want to be with Daddy. Zachary ended up out with Bill, and Buddy fell asleep with me.

Saturday, March 22, 2008

I was feeling much better this morning. My mom called and asked if I wanted her to take Buddy to his scrimmage game. But I felt okay to go. I ended up taking Zachary over there. That way, if I need to go to my car, I can. It was a pretty nice day, and I did fine. After practice, Bill met us at the grocery store. Not only were we overdue, but it didn't help that both Bill and

Buddy were hungry, so you can imagine what our bill was. A funny thing happened while we were there. I ran into a girl that in the past we had our differences and even though I had moved on, she couldn't seem to. Well, today was different, when she saw me she asked me how I was doing? As I was taken by surprise that she even had an interest, I told her I was doing fine. I congratulated her on her newborn and went on my way. Bill had no idea who this girl was, and when she left, I was laughing. He asked, "What's so funny?" I explained who it was and said it is funny that now that I had cancer, she feels the need to be nice to me! Maybe she was thinking back to how she was and realized how silly it was to act that way. Anyway, I am glad that my cancer might have been the reason for another person to realize that life is too short and we need to be as happy as we can be.

I got home, and we unloaded the groceries. We went to Joanne's for dinner and to dye Easter eggs. The kids had a great time, and so did we.

That was quick!

Sunday, March 23, 2008

Happy Easter! The Easter bunny stopped by and hid some eggs. In fact, he hid one so well that we couldn't find it! We went to Joanne's for breakfast, and then we played some games. While we were playing, Darla (my miniature dachshund) jumped on my lap. Joanne said, "Um, I think Darla is having a reaction to something. Look at her face!" Her face was all swollen, and she was getting hives all over her. We jumped up and started calling different animal places. We ended up taking her to Veterinary Specialty Center of Delaware in Newport. What a nice place! Joanne, Jessica, and I took Darla while Brenda cleaned up and Bill and John stayed with the kids. When we got there, some of her swelling and hives had gone away, but we went in anyway. Once we got there, the receptionist called for the triage to come to the front! How cute.

We took her back. They examined her, and they gave her a shot of Benadryl. They thought that she might have been bitten by a bug. This is very common for this time of year.

I was very impressed about the place, so if your animal ever has an emergency, that is the place to go. They said that Darla would be sleepy the rest of the day.

When we got home, the rest of the day was spent getting ready for Easter dinner at Mom and Dad's. I was in charge of the deviled eggs. When I was done, I got a bath. While I was changing my bandage, I noticed that the darn thing is getting bigger! I couldn't wait till Tuesday to see Warren.

The Easter egg hunt at Mom and Dad's was fun, and dinner was delicious. I talked about the last time I had broccoli casserole. It was on Thanksgiving, and I couldn't really taste it since it was during my chemo treatment. Time flies, doesn't it!

We left around half past eight in the evening. A busy, eventful but great day!

Monday, March 24, 2008

Not too much happened today! It is the first day of spring break for the kids. They will be with me since I am off. I guess we didn't do anything too exciting because I can't remember. I did fill out a questionnaire for a study that I am going to be a part of for the HGC. There will be three other couples that will have eight sessions with a psychologist discussing breast cancer and how it has affected us. It should be interesting. I did go to the firehouse, and I was brave and didn't wear anything on my head. Some people say that I look like Jamie Lee Curtis and that I am making a trend with my "white patch." I would feel more comfortable with it being a little bit longer, but I am ready to not wear the scarves anymore, unless it is chilly out.

Tuesday, March 25, 2008

Yeah, it's finally here. I got to see Dr. Warren, but I had to wait till 1:45 for my appointment. Bill was taking some FMLA time to be there with me since we thought this was going to be a decision-making day. We went back, and she asked what has been going on. She laid me back and said that yes, the suture opened again. The whitish layer is again the protein film that has formed. Once she took that away, it was opened underneath and fluid came out. I couldn't see it, but Bill told me what she did. She was examining, and I informed her that I have prepared myself for the news of needing to remove the expander. She pushed a little, much gentler than the on-call doctor would do it and said that this was what she wanted to do: "I want to get you into the surgical room and recontour the tissue."

I have a "lump" of extra tissue towards the middle, and she wanted to sedate me, debride the area even though there was no sign of infection, and cut or pull the good tissue over to cover the opening. The opening, to give you a visual, is about half the size of a dime. So it is not this gaping hole. Now you may understand how we have had healing. We were so close to it being healed so it is depressing to know that it might fail because of this small area. She put some bandage on and told me that we would talk with her scheduling coordinator, Susan, who could work some miracles to get me in this week. Bill and I went and saw Susan, who was on the phone with the surgicenter in Wilmington where Brenda works. Yeah! Well, Susan needs to work on her social skills because she certainly wasn't the friendliest person.

We corrected her that it was my left side and not my right side, and you might have thought we told her that she was ugly or something. She told the person on the phone, "Okay, the husband is telling me it is the left not the right." She then slammed her pen on the counter, stood up, whipped the paper from the printer, and made a copy. You know me; ignore it because she may be having a bad day. So I thanked her for working her miracles and getting me in on Friday. Guess what the response was. "Uh-huh!" NO smile, eye contact. Nothing! So when we went to the front desk, I said to the receptionist, "It takes a lot to make her smile, doesn't it?" Well, I must not be the only one who has commented that because she just smiled and agreed when I said it. She must work a lot of great miracles to be able to keep her job! Bill was good too because he was biting his tongue the whole time we were in with her. Anyway, her miracles got me into the surgicenter on Friday, March 28 at 1:30 p.m. I went over to the HGC to get some blood work, and of course, they were coming over to me telling me to hang in there and that I look great! I then went to my radiologist and informed Karen that I will not be starting radiation on Friday because I am getting minor surgery. She scheduled me for two weeks out, which puts me on April 11 for a re-evaluation to see if I will need to get a new CAT scan. If there is much tissue contour change, then we will have to rescan. Otherwise, we can use the same one, and they can work on the angle and whatever else they do to set me up for radiation. Then out walked Strasser, and he said, "So now she is deciding to do surgery?"

I said, "Yes, and she knows that you are getting impatient with her."

He said, "Well, it is a good thing I am going through my anger management classes right now. Just let her know that I don't have any guns or weapons on me!"

He is a jokester. Why can't more people be that way? Maybe he should talk to Susan!

So we left, and when I got home, I made my phone calls. I waited till I got home since my cell phone has gotten a lot of use this month, but that made my mom and Joanne worry that much more. Sorry! I did call Brenda on my cell so that she could get a heads-up and work on my anesthesiologist team.

That night, we had some people over from our Relay for Life team and talked about our Beef-and-Beer we are having on April 18 to raise money for ACS. It sounds like we are going to have a good turnout, and I am looking forward to it.

Wednesday, March 26, 2008

It was a busy day on the road. Joanne dropped off Zachary since it is picture day at preschool. I dropped off Jaylyn at her babysitter's, headed back home, and got ready for our busy day. Buddy, Jessica, and I went to pick up Zachary; and we all headed to my office for them to get their teeth cleaned. All went well. Buddy has a chip on a back tooth, and decay is underneath it. So he is the lucky one who needs to come back for his first filling. It is on a baby tooth, but he will have it for a while, so we will fill it. He also needs sealants. We then went to get some lunch, and I dropped Jessica and Zachary at Joanne's work while Buddy and I went to see Dr. Luft for his ears. As soon as Dr. Luft looked in his ears, he said, "Oh, definite fluid in the right ear and some on the left, but not as much."

If you put your fingers in your ears and talk, this is what it sounds like for Buddy! Dr. Luft did all kinds of things to his nose and checked his adenoids. It was pretty interesting. He told us that he would like to put tubes in his ears, take out his adenoids, and shave his tonsils. The tonsil part is an option, but he said that later on he will probably need to have that done. This is not a surgery that has to be done immediately, but we would like to get it done soon. With the tonsils, he will miss five days of school. Without the tonsils done, he might miss one day of school. We left without making an appointment because if you schedule an appointment and then cancel, you will be charged a very big sum because they are holding operating room time.

After the appointment, I came up with more questions and knew that I will have to call and ask. I was relieved in a way that it has not been just our imagination that he has had problems with his hearing. But on the other hand, I feel bad that this has been going on for so long. We went back to pick up Zachary and Jessica and then went to pick up their cousin Victoria. We went home to get some snacks and headed off to baseball practice. Buddy ended up having a friend come over for the night. As I lay in bed, I was feeling pretty good and looking forward to Friday.

Thursday, March 27, 2008

Joanne had a therapy appointment, so I opened up the day care for the day. I kept Zachary home, so he could enjoy the fun. There were six kids here. You know, after three, who's counting? Everyone had a good day and an active one. I got some cleaning done to prepare for tomorrow, and Joanne made sure the kids told her if I lifted anything heavy. I was a good girl although the temptation was there.

—

All of the kids went home; mine stayed with me, of course. Bill did not get off until ten in the evening since he was going to his second job at the 9-1-1 center when he gets off at the plant. He is such a hard worker. I feel bad that he works so much, but he doesn't seem to mind most of the time.

It was nine in the evening, and I ate some ice cream. I tried to stay awake, but I was out right after that.

More interesting times!

Friday, March 28, 2008

I woke up at six thirty in the morning and knew that I had to finish my updates for you. No one was awake, so I headed to the computer and started typing away. I took a break to fix the kids' breakfast, but they slept in till nine in the morning since they did have a busy day yesterday. Bill was taking Zachary to school, and Buddy will be with Joanne. I have taken my Tamoxifen and had my little bit of water. Now I have to stay away from the kitchen because all I am seeing is food. It was going to be a long morning. We would be leaving around eleven thirty in the morning to be there by noon. My surgery was at 1:30 p.m. It should take about one hour, and then I will be sent home. Bill will be with me tonight, and my cousin is going to spend the day with me tomorrow. Bill and his best friend Paul are going to New York for the night. Paul's wife asked a while back if Bill would take Paul away for a night. She has been noticing him getting a little stressed. It couldn't have come at a better time because I think Bill needs some time also. He was going to cancel, and I made sure that he didn't. He deserves some downtime too.

I was getting out of the shower when the phone rang. It was the surgicenter, asking if I could come in earlier. I am not sure if they realized what time it was because we were planning on leaving at eleven thirty to be there on time, and they called at 11:10 a.m. Oh well, we headed up there, and when we got into the parking space, I got unbuckled. I must have turned a little too much because I had a gusher. Of course, I didn't put too much padding on since I was about to have surgery. I scared Bill because I was like "Oh my gosh!" You know, it is a very startling feeling when you feel something warm going down your belly!

Anyway, we walked in, and I was holding my left "breast" (you know, like you have a broken arm, and you keep it up to your chest). I checked in, and the receptionist, of course knows Brenda. So we were joking with her, and I asked how long it will be due to my gusher. She said that the patient ahead of me never showed up so they are running on time. She said the doctor will be out shortly, and I told her, "In that case, take me back now! (I was joking, of course).

As we were sitting out there waiting, they gave Bill his name tag and my case number so he will know when I am in the operating room and when I am in the recovery room. This brought back some flashbacks for him from the initial surgery. He said that that was the hardest part, the waiting. Luckily, this one wouldn't be long. They took me back, and everyone couldn't believe how I am so much like Brenda—my looks, demeanor, and voice. I had two ladies checking me and doing my vitals. Then the anesthesiologist came in and got the IV started. Here we go again. She found nothing in the elbow crease and went right for the hand, near the ring finger. She told me that she was going to get me numb prior to inserting the IV. Well, the needle for the numbing was dull, and she had to really work to get it in. But she did a great job. It sounds worse than it was.

Brenda came in and helped me get changed and take my jewelry off. I know that you are not supposed to wear any. But heck, if I don't, people may think I am a man! Bill came back and wished me good luck and gave me a kiss. The nurse put an X on the left "breast," and then Dr. Warren came in and put her initials on it as well. Anyone else want to give me their autograph! This is a new procedure so that there is no question on which side they are working on. They wheeled me back in this recliner chair, pretty nice. Brenda would be in there during the whole procedure. When we got in the room, the nurses were saying hello. Of course, I couldn't really recognize them with their gear on, but it was nice knowing that everyone knows you. Kind of a safe feeling.

I was freezing! I moved over to the operating table, and they put a warm blanket on me. Anne also forewarned me that she was going to put an ice pack on my thigh to ground me! Whatever, all I know is that it was COLD! As I am lying there, I said, "She just put something in the IV, didn't she?"

"Yes."

"It sounds different."

"How does it sound, loud or soft?"

"Oh it sounds soft."

Brenda looked at me and said, "Let's just take these glasses off now." When she took them off, I pretended to pass out. Then I really did because the next thing I remember is hearing them talking and opening my eyes and seeing the blue tarp. I thought to myself, *I wonder if they know that I am awake. I will try to listen to their conversation.* And then before you know it, I was saying hello to them. Some time passed in between there because Warren was suturing up in the beginning, and next, everything was bandaged up. Sedation is great!

They were finished, and all went really well. I thanked everyone before I left, and they wheeled me to the recovery room. I was feeling good, and they wanted me to get some fluids in me prior to leaving. Dr. Warren went to get Bill, went over what we did, and gave instructions. I have a drain again, will take an antibiotic, and have Percocet if needed. I will see her in seven to ten days.

Brenda brought her coworkers in for me to meet, and one of them recently completed her treatments for breast cancer. She is still wearing a wig, but I think she has more hair than me! Since I didn't have my surgery cap on, they all saw my hair. They liked it even with the grey! I think Brenda's friend will remove her wig after today.

I took a Percocet prior to leaving, and then we headed home. We picked up Zachary, stopped by Taco Bell, and went to get my prescriptions. Later at night, Bill took Buddy and Zachary to baseball practice, and I got some shuteye.

Oh, but before I forget, I have to tell you a funny story. You know how I am concerned with the chin/face hair, right? Well, I used to get the occasional black hairs on my chin. Since the hair was gone, I hadn't been checking. Joanne and I were on our way to Middletown last week, and we were at a red light. I can't remember if Joanne saw a black hair or I happened to look in the visor mirror, when OH MY GOSH, I not only had one, but I had five, yes five black hairs coming out. I am such a Chewbacca. I went to working on getting those things with my fingers. How embarrassing. I frequently check myself now, and I carry tweezers in my purse!

Saturday, March 29, 2008

Bill headed off to New York at five thirty in the morning. My cousin Sherri spent the day with me. It was a great day. The kids played wonderfully together, and Sherri and I had some quality time spent together. She had lunch and dinner for me. It was MUCH appreciated. Her hubby came over and took Buddy to baseball practice for me. They left about eight in the evening, and then Joanne came and took over. I have taken some Percocet throughout the day, and it controlled the discomfort.

Sunday, March 30, 2008

I hope not to have to take any Percocet today. Since Bill has left, he has called about every ten minutes to check and make sure that I am okay. I reassure him that I am doing okay and tell him to enjoy himself.

The firehouse had an Easter egg hunt today, and my friend Michelle Smith came over to taxi us to and from. The kids had a good time, and I felt okay. But I kept my distance from everyone for fear of getting hit or bumped. After a very eventful time with the kids, Michelle brought us back to the house. She wanted to make sure that I didn't need anything else and told me to call if she could do anything else to help me. Friends, along with family, are a wonderful thing.

We went to Joanne's for dinner, and Bill got home about seven thirty in the evening. He had a really good time, and I am glad that he was able to get away. The kids were very happy to see him and fill him in on what we did.

Monday, March 31, 2008

Not too much happened this day. Brenda did call me and tell me that her coworker came in today without her wig on. She said that I am an inspiration to her. I am so happy to help people.

I took it easy, and no Percocet was needed. I felt pain every now and then but not enough that I needed to take something. Buddy saw Ms. Kym (psychiatrist) today, and it was a good meeting. She said he opened up today on how he had been acting at school and towards his cousin. She gave him some suggestions to try. You know it is so hard because they don't go into detail on what they said. This is not only because of confidentiality but also because of trust. If she did tell me everything and then I talked to Buddy about it, then what would the reason be in seeing her? Buddy wouldn't feel he could open up if he knew that she told me what he said. Anyway, it went well.

Tuesday, April 1, 2008

I found out that I am pregnant! April fool's! Really, there is no chance of that happening right now. I just thought that I would give you a jaw-dropper.

HA-HA! I thought that I had an appointment with Warren to get the drain out, but it is tomorrow. So I got another uneventful day. Yeah! But I need to get ready for tomorrow.

Wednesday, April 2, 2008

Bill was off and would be with me today for my visits. I met with Dr. Hazuda to discuss when I will be returning. I also have my appointment with Warren. It was one thirty in the afternoon, and we were off to see Dr. Hazuda. I was giving him my resignation. I have thought really long and really hard about this and have decided that I am not going back. I have definitely had a major change in my life, and I see things differently. I see how important it is for my kids that I am home when they get off of the bus and help them with their homework, have dinner, and get them to their activities without having to rush around and not be able to spend some quality time with them. It is very hard for me to give my resignation because I have been with Dr. H for fourteen years. And not only am I going to miss my coworkers, but I am deeply going to miss my patients who have really become my friends. You have to understand that when patients come to see me, they not only get their teeth cleaned, but we would have psychiatry session at times—for them and me. Do you know how good it is to talk to someone who doesn't really know your family and friends, and you can just let it out to someone? It feels good, and I saw that with a lot of my patients. I am sure that they saw that with me. Anyway, I had all intentions on going back, but after realizing how important this is to me and knowing that I will be out for another forty-five days plus, I felt it was time to let Dr. H know of my decision. So, we got there, and of course, I was showing off my hair. No scarf or hat anymore. I got a hug from a patient. She was unaware of my situation and wished me luck. Dr. H and Julie (his wife) saw the hair for the first time. Dr. H said, "I didn't realize you had that much grey!"

"Yeah, me neither, that is why I colored it." Oh well, the truth is out now. We went back to his office, and I told him of my decision. He was speechless. He asked me if I am not going to work at all, and I told him that I do not plan on stopping hygiene altogether, but I can no longer work till five in the afternoon, and I don't want to have the long drive (Middletown to Pike Creek). To my surprise, he told me that he is not going to accept my resignation! WHAT! He told me that we have too long of a relationship to just call it quits. He accepted my resignation for my current position but not for the office completely. He told me to do what I have to do with treatment, and then afterwards, we will reevaluate my situation and see if we can work something out. He didn't want me to take any of my personal items with me until we meet later. I feel sorry for the person who will replace me; she is going to feel like she is mourning me with my pictures still there. Anyway, in reality, the only thing that we could really work out is my working there on Wednesdays for my hours because there is no room for another hygienist any other day. So that may be a possibility. That way, I can still see some of my patients.

As I came out of the office, Bill saw that I was smiling and not crying and thought that it wasn't what he expected. Well, me neither. I had letters to all of my coworkers, explaining what I was doing and why. Debbie, our front desk staff, had tears in her eyes when I told her what I had done. I didn't want to bother the other girls, and I also had to get to another appointment. Bill said, "Geez you can't even quit your job!" I tell them that I will keep in touch with them, and then we headed out.

We were off to Warren's to get my drain out—or not. When we got there and she saw how much I have been draining (written on my log), she suggested keeping the drain in. She did not want to take the chance of fluid building up and breaking open the stitch. Fine by me! So all in all, this was a wash-out day. I didn't really accomplish anything that I ventured to do.

Later that night, Bill took Buddy to baseball practice, and Zachary and I stayed home and played.

Thursday, April 3, and Friday, April 4, 2008

Not too much happened these days. I am limited to what I can do because I do not want anything to open. Needless to say, the house is not really getting cleaned right now, but I manage to occupy my time in other ways.

Saturday, April 5, 2008

We got Buddy to practice by eleven in the morning, and Joanne kept Zachary. You know, it is so hard to find something to wear when you have this drain hanging off the side of your "breast." And it hangs all the way down past your shirts. I have to do some creative pinning so no one can see it. Black is always a good color for this. We take one of Buddy's friends home, and he ended up staying there for a little while. When I got home, Joanne was planning on going to a jewelry party. There was going to be a guy there who will buy your gold jewelry. So I went through my jewelry box and saw what I can give him. We headed to the party, and I had some old necklaces, bracelets, and charms. The jewelry that this girl makes is really nice, but I didn't get anything today. What I do get is $340 for my gold! Sweet. When do you go to a party and you get money (cash)?

We were running a little late because I needed to get home and get ready for a wedding that the Ladies Auxiliary are serving for, and I still had to pick up Buddy. When I got home, I got the mail, and Buddy has gotten honor roll. YEAH! I finally got Buddy and went to the firehouse. All went well, but this dag on drain is in the way. But I know it needs to be there.

Sunday, April 6, 2008

Not too much happened today. I did go to my mom's for takeout—meatloaf, my favorite. The boys have had a little bit of a listening problem today, and I figured it was best that they aren't around my parents. Besides, my mom has a pretty nasty cold. Dinner was delicious.

Well, it was time for bed, and guess what? Yep, you guessed it, I have a peeping hole! What the heck! I called Brenda and told her that I see a small opening starting. It was really small. I will see Dr. Warren tomorrow. Brenda asked what I have been doing, but really, I haven't done anything to overwork myself. I informed Bill when he called, but he tried to reassure me that it will be fine. I covered the site and went to bed.

Monday, April 7, 2008

I checked the spot, and it has gotten a little bigger overnight. My appointment with Warren was at 8:45 a.m., and my friend Kathy is coming with me. Bill was going to get Buddy to school. He was just getting off of night work, and I wanted him to get some sleep.

Dr. Warren came in and asked, "Well, how are we doing?"

I told her that we have a peeper trying to come out. She looked at it and said that she may not do anything because she doesn't know how many layers have formed, and since the drain was still keeping suction, then it was "closed." But when I told her that it had gotten bigger overnight, and then she got the Q-tip and started cleaning around it. And yep, we are open! What was surprising was that the drain was keeping suction with the opening. It didn't hurt when she cleaned it. It was seeing her moving it around and knowing what she was doing. Kathy had to turn away for this part. Speaking of which, it was pretty funny when she asked me when we got in the room if I wanted her to turn around while I got changed. Ha, are you kidding?

Like you haven't seen this before. Dignity is out the window. These really aren't my breasts; they are just uneven mounds right now. Anyway, she was surprised to see how great the right side looks, and now she has an actual visual when I am explaining what my opening looks like. We definitely got some laughs during the whole process, and I can't tell you how great it is to have a bosom buddy with you who has gone or is going through the same thing. Some people just would not get our sense of humor. Anyway, Dr. Warren came in, got me numb and stitched the heck out of me. We kept the drain in, and she explained that where it opened is where all of the skin was pulled together and that it can happen. Of course, I would be the one that it would happen to. She wanted to see me in a couple of days to check on things. I made my appointment, and we left.

Afterwards, Kathy and I went to the HGC, and I went ahead and cancelled my appointment with Strasser. I told Karen, his nurse, that I was going to have to cancel for Friday since I knew that I was going to be "sick" that day! Out came Strasser, and he was holding up his hand, saying, "I am going to pretend like I can't see you!" He has such a great sense of humor. I proceeded to tell them what was really going on, and we rescheduled the CAT scan for next Friday, April 18. Kathy and I left and headed to breakfast at Guilday's on Route 40. It looked like a dive, but it was good!

I can explain to you how our chemo brain works. During our adventures, Kathy would walk passed my van every time, because she just forgot. When we are talking, we have to help each other out because we forget certain words that we are trying to say. And another thing, Brenda had told me before that it is good to have another set of ears at my doctor's appointments since I seem to forget so easily. Well, I guess having another chemo brain with me doesn't help too much, but we have fun trying to remember. Scary thought, isn't it?

On my way to breakfast, I called Brenda to tell her what Dr. Warren said and did. She was flustered. She had just gotten a phone call from Dave, and he had informed her that his convoy had been hit but that no one was hurt. If we heard it on the news. We shouldn't worry, he is okay. He only has a little over a month, and it can't come soon enough. So, continued prayers for his safe return are requested.

Later that night, Buddy and I took Zachary to his first baseball game of the season. It was freezing out there; I am ready for the warm weather. I am not in any discomfort, but just on the cautious side with everything I do.

Tuesday, April 8, 2008

I went to Buddy's school to volunteer for the day. Ms. Phillips is always so appreciative of my time. I enjoy being there. I will enjoy every minute of it since I know that Buddy will not want me around soon enough. The kids were asking me about my hair: "Why did you cut your hair so short?" "Were you sick, is that why you don't have hair?" My favorite question: "What is that white spot?" I answered them all, and we got on to schoolwork. Later, Bill took Buddy to practice, and Zachary went with me to Cub Scouts. We were getting ready for the cub mobile, and the kids were painting their car.

Everything is still intact, and I continue to keep my fingers crossed that nothing opens.

Wednesday, April 9, 2008

I didn't have any doctor's appointments today, and I hung out at the house. That night, I had a Volunteer Appreciation Dinner to go to at Michael's restaurant. This is given by the Colonial Education Association, and Ms. Phillips gave them my name. They handed out certificates to the parents who volunteered. It was very nice, and I met a lot of nice people. I unfortunately missed Buddy's first game, but Bill told me that he did really well.

Thursday, April 10, 2008

I saw Dr. Warren at 10:30 a.m., and it was nice and quick. Everything is still closed, and she still wanted to keep the drain in for security purposes. That is all right with me. She wanted to see me early next week, but the only thing that she had was on Thursday. I hoped for a cancellation to get in earlier, but we all know how that goes.

I went to do some errands and then I stopped at the Doghouse to pick up some lunch for Bill and I. When I got home, I learned that he has been mulching all morning. He took a break to sit out on the deck and have some lunch. You gotta love those kinds of moments. After that, it was off to working again for him.

Today is my friend Melinda's and her husband Todd's anniversary, and I hope they got to enjoy the day or evening. Happy Anniversary.

Friday, April 11, 2008

Not too much happened this day either, but don't you worry, I thought of something to do. I was having my friends' kids over tonight. My friend was meeting me at Buddy's practice. While I was at Caravel where the boys practice, I ran into a patient of mine. She was surprised to hear my news and understood the whole being-with-the-kids thing. She has four kids herself, and she was there watching two of her kids' softball games. She wished me luck and held back her tears!

When we got home, the kids played for a little while and had a great time with each other. Bill finally got the kids off to sleep, and we got ready for our busy ball day tomorrow.

Saturday, April 12, 2008

We had opening day today for ball, pictures, and games. We decided not to go to the opening ceremonies and instead hang around the house and play. We headed to the ball field, and it was a busy day. I ran into so many people who have not seen me in a while, and I explained how I am doing. It was like a reunion. I went capless, so more people saw my hair. Most people said that they like it and it looks like I frosted it. We'll see how it goes if I even color it again. You know me, plain Jane. Pictures went smoothly for the boys, and we had one and a half hours to play on the playground and get a snack. The problem started when both boys had a game at four thirty in the afternoon. I had to split my time up. Buddy understood that I needed to be with Zachary the majority of the time but that I would continue to check on him. Zachary was in coach's pitch and hit a "homerun," but with the little guys, you can't go all the way home. He ran right past his teammate who was on second base. We then went to watch Buddy, and I missed him pitch. But I saw him make an out on third and get up to bat a couple of times. He is in kid pitch and he is starting to like pitching! We were supposed to go to an end-of-the-season wrestling party, but the kids told me that they didn't want to go. Instead, we hung out at home and then went to Dairy Queen. Bill had been craving a hot fudge sundae.

As I got myself ready for bed, I changed my dressing, and I noticed a little opening. But not to worry! It is different than the other openings that I have had. It is the size of a pinhead, and there is not a stitch around it. I was thinking that it is healing from the inside out, and I will see if it gets bigger in the morning.

Sunday, April 13, 2008

My mom, Buddy, Zachary, myself and others from the firehouse went to Medieval Times in Baltimore. We were given tickets by a very good friend of ours who could not make it, and they did not want the tickets to go to waste. It was very generous of them, and it was much appreciated. The kids had a blast, and my mom had just as much fun. She told me that I had to stop yelling/cheering because she was afraid that I might rip a stitch.

Monday, April 14 and Tuesday, April 15, 2008

Not too much went on. The good news is that the hole has not gotten any bigger. I am keeping myself busy with getting ready for the Beef-and-Beer this Friday. We are selling out, and things are coming together. I have doctor's appointments for the rest of the week. Wednesday is my first-three-months check with Dr. Biggs. Not really sure what he will do or say, but I am hoping it is all good. Thursday is with Dr. Warren, and I am hopeful that the drain and some stitches will come out. Friday is with Dr. Strasser, and this will hopefully be my re-CAT scan. Radiation will start next week.

As always, I want you to remember how important friends and family are. You never realize how many you have until something like this comes along. I thank all of you for your support, cards, and prayers.

Time To Throw In The Towel!

Wednesday, April 16, 2008

I started my day out with making phone calls to the person who said she would donate all of the food for our Beef-and-Beer. She said that we would meet on Wednesday night to get the food. Long story short, I called six to seven times throughout the day, and days passed, and there was no return phone call. Looks like I have been stood up.

I had my first-three-month check up with Dr. Biggs. He just asked me some questions and checked my vitals. Pretty uneventful, which is a good thing. I, of course, had some questions: "Out of all of the different kinds of breast cancers, how serious was mine?" He never gave me a straight answer but did tell me that there are many people out there whose conditions are more serious. Ya don't say!

"Is there any certain test that you can do to see if you have gotten all of the cancer?"

"No. If I had a scan that could go over your entire body, that would be great. But there is none. There are tests that we can do, but there are more false positives, so they just go by clinical signs."

Pretty scary, huh? Bill wasn't there, but he doesn't agree with this at all and says that he wants some kind of test done. So I told him that he could call Dr. Biggs and discuss it with him. There are two ways to look at this: (1) You don't want to go the rest of your life taking tests to see if you have cancer; but (2) if you wait till the clinical signs show, won't you take the chance of it being harder to treat? It is something to think about. Anyway,

---

he didn't say too much when I said that I hadn't had my radiation yet, and then he said that he would check me in three months.

Since my appointment was at 3:40 p.m., Bill didn't go with me. He was home for Buddy. We had tickets to the Blue Rocks game. Buddy got two tickets for reading ten books, and we got the other two from a friend who was giving them away. (We have been pretty lucky with that). Bill is going into work late so that he can make the game. The kids had a great time, but it was a little brisk sitting out there. You could tell who I brought because Zachary and I were prepared. Bill and Buddy, on the other hand, had on shorts and were cold. As my Dad always said, "You can always take off, but you can never put on if you don't have it."

Thursday, April 17, 2008

Since I never heard back from the girl from the food source, I now have a mission of purchasing all of the food for tomorrow. I work well under pressure. I have a 10:00 a.m. appointment with Warren. She saw the opening and decided that she didn't want to do anything with it. Down towards the bottom of the site, it was pretty red. She didn't think that it is infected, but she put me on an antibiotic just in case. This is also another reason she left that area alone. She didn't want to "stir" anything up if there was infection. She also wanted to continue to leave the drain in since I am still getting about forty CC's a day. She would like to see it below thirty. Also, since there is a slight opening, we didn't want to take the drain out and take the chance of it building up and opening more. Her concern with leaving the drain in is that it may be causing irritation on the bottom. We don't want that tissue to "go bad." I would hate to be a doctor. I don't feel there is a right or wrong way of doing it but more of a chance that you make the right decision. So, I left with my drain and my prescription. She wants to see me next week.

I headed right over to Strasser to let him know that I still have the drain in. They couldn't do the CAT scan with that in, so we cancelled my appointment for tomorrow. They teased me while I was there, but then we decided that I will just call them after I get my drain out. Maybe this will change my luck, and I can get to movin'!"

Off to purchase the items for tomorrow. It really wasn't that bad; the Ladies' Auxiliary had the beef and green beans. I had to get the rest. At night, my dad took Zachary to his game. We met down at the firehouse to set up and prepare for the Beef-and-Beer. The hall looked great, and Bill and I are very thankful for all who have helped out.

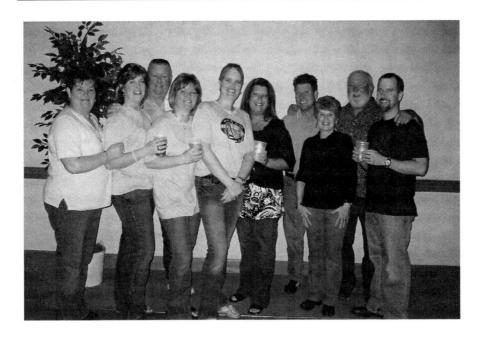

Sutton Family and Reynolds Family at the 1st
Annual Team Survivor Beef and Beer

Friday, April 18, 2008

Since I had no doctor's appointments, I got to spend the morning down at the firehouse getting the beef and coleslaw ready for tonight. We were expecting over two hundred people! I went home and finished my T-shirt that has our Relay for Life team logo on the front and the word "SURVIVOR" on the back. We got the boys ready to take to our friend's house, and off we went for the night.

I can't explain the fun we had. I saw so many people whom I had not seen in such a long time. It was like a big reunion. We did run out of beef and green beans around eight thirty in the evening, but that was an hour after the food was first put out. I didn't hear any complaints about that since really it wasn't about the food but for the cause. It was so nice to see my parents on the floor, dancing and having a good time together. Now, for those of you who left on the early side, you missed a monumental moment. My mom, who hardly ever drinks, had a little too much Captain Morgan, Jell-O shooters, and I think even a test tube shot! Later in the evening, someone brought out a pole, and people were dancing on it and around it. I was at the bar, getting a soda. You know me, I don't need alcohol to have a good time, and

I saw someone on the floor. I asked my friend Cheryl who that was, and she said, "Your mother!" Yes, that is right; my mom was on the floor WITH the pole. She apparently was lured out by my hubby and then he quickly turned around and left her out there by herself. She obviously didn't care at that point, and she thought that the pole was attached to the floor (how, I have no idea). She grabbed a hold of it, and they both went down. That didn't stop her. She got up and still gave us some laughs! My sister did get it on video, and we keep telling her we are going to put it on You Tube! I think after that, Mom was ready to go home. Most people left around eleven in the evening. We had said, "Isn't it funny how our lives change? Ten years ago, we would have been here till two in the morning, and we would have seen where we could go for breakfast. But now, we have kids and jobs that we need to attend to. I do hope that we get to do this again next year, but I am pretty sure that you won't see my mom on the pole again!

When we got home, Bill and I counted to see how much money we raised. We counted around $4,600! We are very excited to be able to have this go to cancer research. I did feel bad, and we made an announcement because a good amount of people thought that the fundraiser was for me specifically. I totally appreciate all of the support we had. Bill and I definitely have had a change of life, but financially we are doing okay. Of course, everyone would love to have more money, but right now we are "surviving."

Before I went to bed, I of course change my dressing. I noticed that my drain lost its suction, from too much dancing maybe. I reclosed it. I heard a slight whistle, and pop, there goes the suction again. Houston, we have sprung a leak! I looked at the site and noticed another little area. Now, most of you may think that it was related to the dancing, but I reassure you that it is not. I closed it up with some Bacitracin. The suction stayed and, I went off to bed.

Saturday, April 19, 2008

My suction is still there. Yeah! We had to go pick up Buddy at eight in the morning for a game at nine. Boy am I glad that I didn't drink last night. We ran into a friend of ours who was there last night. Put it this way, it looked like it was going to be a long day for him!

After the game, we headed home and waited to leave for Zachary's game. I checked my suction, and some air has gotten in. I didn't have a good feeling about it. I closed it again and went on my way. My friend brought Zachary home, and he said that his belly was really hurting. He was very pale. So, no baseball game for him today. He lay down, and Pam and I just hung out and had a relaxing time together. What I am trying to say is that I wasn't doing much of anything in hopes that my suction stays and nothing gets bigger. FAT CHANCE! Does anyone have a clue yet on why I named this update the way that I did? If not, it will come soon enough. Suspense, you gotta love it. Oh yeah, an update on my mom. She has been sitting on a heating pad all day, and she has been talking to "Ben Gay"!

Sunday, April 20, 2008

I pretty much did nothing. Bill took off from the 9-1-1 center to be home with the boys. It was an off-and-on rainy day. The boys ended up playing with the neighbor, but I was glad that Bill was home. I told Buddy that his assembly is going to be held tomorrow, and he told me that I didn't have to go. I asked him if he was embarrassed of me, and he very quickly said NO! Just thought that I would ask, but I am still going. My mom is still having a little lower back discomfort, so I don't think she will be doing much of anything either. When I changed my dressing, I did notice that the area seems to be getting bigger! Oh H!@# ! I applied more Bacitracin and covered it up.

Monday, April 21, 2008

Yep, I think I am going to have to see Warren sooner. Suction is staying, but I don't like the looks of it. I have an Honor Roll assembly to go to for Buddy. He is eight years old, and he is already starting to not want to sit with me! I saw some kids from his class but no Buddy. I looked around the room, and there he was, sitting with some of his classmates. He waved to me, and the assembly started. When I looked over, I noticed that he was sitting next to a girl, Hazel, and I think that would be his reason for not wanting to sit next to me. Oh my gosh, not already!

The assembly was nice, and when we left, I made a phone call to Dr. Warren's office. She was done for the morning, and I can get in tomorrow at nine thirty in the morning. I decided to go home and have another do-nothing kind of day. Which, I have to tell you, I CAN'T STAND! It makes my family feel good, but it is very hard for me.

Zachary had a game later that night, and again he loved hitting the ball. The outfield is what we need to work on, but for a five-year-old he's not bad. As for my mom, she continues to use the heating pad and says she is making an appointment to see the doctor (how will you explain to the Doctor how this happened ?).

———

Tuesday, April 22, 2008

I looked at the site and noticed that the area isn't as red, but the opening seems to continue to get bigger. What started out as a small pinhead is now the size of an elongated pea. If you can picture that. I don't want you to think that I have this gaping hole because I know that when I mention an opening, you may think big.

I dropped the kids off, and I pretty much prepared myself for these words: "We are going to have to remove the expander." I waited for Dr. Warren, and as soon as she came in, we pretty much could read each other's mind. She looked at the area and said, "Okay, we've come to a point when we are going to have to make a decision. We need to get you started on your radiation treatment, and this isn't cooperating." I told her that I pretty much expected it and prepared myself for her to say that. She said she could tell by the look on my face. So, she wants to remove the expander, get the radiation, let me heal, and then talk about reconstruction. She said that she could remove it in the office. It wouldn't hurt, but it would be uncomfortable. Yeah, let's not go there. She gave me the option of keeping the drain in or taking out. If I take it out, I could get some leakage, so I opted to leave it in. She apologized to me, and I told her that there was no need because it is not her fault. She did everything that she could to try and save it. I just wish that we could have proved everyone wrong. So I went to schedule another surgery for Friday, April 25 at 10:45 a.m. She is also going to take my port out of my arm since I won't need that anymore! When I left the office, I got on the phone and made all of my phone calls. I started the conversation out with "Well, we have lost the battle!" (I didn't want to put that as the subject because I didn't want you to get scared that the cancer was back.) Everyone wanted to know how I am doing, and I think that since I already had my cry when the on-call doctor had told me, I had prepared myself for this to happen. I spoke to my "boobie buddy" Kathy last, and she reassured me on my thoughts. I sat there and thought "did I make the right decision?". Should I have gotten a double mastectomy? Should I have only gotten a single and went for the Tram to begin with? I almost got myself down about it, thinking of failing. But then I remember "to joke is to cope." So during my conversation with Kathy, I said that I am just going to be a spokesperson on breast cancer reconstructive procedures. Think about it, when all this is said and done, I may have tried all of them—mastectomy, chemo, radiation (eventually), expanders, implants (eventually), prosthesis, tram flap (possible). Bring it on, and I will be able to say, "Yep, I did that too!"

—

The rest of my day was kind of somber, but I got through it. We later went to Buddy's ball game and came home to call it a night.

As for my mom, she went to the doctor and got an X-ray of her lower back to make sure nothing is broken. She just told the doctor it was from dancing. She didn't happen to mention about the pole.

Wednesday, April 23, 2008

I was supposed to go to Buddy's school today, but he informed me that he wanted me to come tomorrow since he is reading to the kindergarteners today, and there won't be much for me to do. So, I guess I will do that tomorrow. I hung out at Zachary's school for a little bit, and then I went for a nice three-mile walk at the park on Route 40. I came home and got started on my update. I have a viewing to go to for my close friend Lisa whose dad passed away from Parkinson's. So if you could have her and her family in your prayers.

I did speak to my mom, and there was no word from the doctor. But she said that today, she has not had to use the heating pad, and she is ready to go again. Yeah right!

Now that you are updated on my happenings, here is a little update on my feelings. You might get the tissues ready, as I have been told that some of you who read my updates get a little emotional. During this whole process, I have been very positive and feel great. I still am, but I am normal, and some of those times, what I'm thinking of aren't happy thoughts but sad ones. I am very happy to say that I found the lump and that we got things moving along. Did I catch it soon enough? Time will tell. Did I make the right decisions? Who will ever know? Is all of the cancer gone? Who knows? But that is not going to stop me from living my life to the fullest. If it returns, there is nothing that I can do about it but fight it again. I look at my family and often think what it would be like if I wasn't here. I know it is a bad thought, but I am just being honest. Last night when we were in bed, Bill asked me if reading "Hanging Out with Lab Coats" (for the second time) made me sad. I told him no and that I can relate to how she felt and what she went through. I told him that I am not afraid, and that if I died, I died (I didn't mean for it to come out like this). What I mean is that I am not thinking of dying, but we all know that whether it is cancer, a car accident, Parkinson's, we could and will all die sometime, so I am not going to say that I haven't thought about it. But until then, we need to enjoy our life and what we have. Bill shared with me that he is scared and notices that he gets agitated very easily since my diagnosis. I know that our relationship is a very strong one, and we are here to help each other out. We will fight this, no doubt. I just like making things challenging! So with that said, I don't want you to think that I am giving up by any means. I just know that I haven't shared some of my thoughts with you, and some of you want to know but don't know how to ask. I continue to be positive and upbeat and can't wait for the celebration when this is all done!

I again want to thank all of you who have contributed to the Relay for Life, attended the Beef-and-Beer (or just purchased tickets), read my updates, and kept me in your thoughts and prayers. I hope that I did not upset anyone with my last paragraph. I do not want you to worry about me. As I have told you before, my updates are very therapeutic for me, and it is my way of remembering ten years from now just how I was feeling!

It Feels Good!
(And Weird)

Thursday, April 24, 2008

I spent all day at Buddy's school volunteering. I had my list of duties to do, and I thoroughly enjoyed it. As usual, the kids were happy to see me. I didn't even sit next to Buddy at lunch because the other kids wanted to sit next to me. Gee, I feel like the popular "kid" in school.

I informed the boys that I will be getting another surgery. Even though they understand that term, they don't seem to have that much of an external reaction, but that is okay. I stopped eating around nine in the evening and got ready for bed. I have taken some pictures of my "breast" during this process. I wish that I would have taken some at the earlier stages, but I certainly don't want to go back so I can get them. Anyway, I am taking them for my purposes; it is amazing how quickly you can forget what things looked like. When I look back at some of the pictures, I think to myself, *Oh my gosh, remember that?* Now I just have to figure out who would develop them, although when you look at them, you can't really tell that it is a "breast"!

Friday, April 25, 2008

Today was another surgery day and Bill was going to cut grass all day so that he can be home all day tomorrow. Even though it was killing him not being there for me, it was the better thing to do. Mom took me today. I asked her to stop by Dunkin' Donuts and pick up some munchkins for my "team" today. Thank goodness, my surgery is earlier in the day, not as long of a wait for fasting. Buddy was off to school, and Zachary spent the night with Aunt Doe Doe. I got my shower, and while I was drying off, I noticed that a white piece of the drain was showing. So I gently pushed it back in. But I also noticed that there are holes in this white part and that my suction was no longer holding. Perfect timing! I, like last time, didn't put as much dressing on since I was about to have surgery. By the way, the holes are where the fluid goes in to fill the drainage ball. When we got to the exit to the hospital, I was feeling a drip on my side where the drain is. I checked, no big deal, keep driving. When we got into the parking lot, déjà vu happened, I got a much bigger drip down my side. I asked Mom if she had any tissues, and she gave me one that has Vicks on it. Oh great. I tried not to touch it too close to the site, not that there is enough on the tissue to do anything, but with me, you never know. Brenda was calling us when we were in the parking lot, and I filled her in. She told me to come in, and she would give me some gauze. On my way in there, I ran into my cousin's husband. His daughter was getting some surgery on her feet. It was a family gathering. I went to check in, and Brenda gave me some gauze. I registered and then I had to sit a little while this time. They were pretty busy today. Brenda would periodically come out to give us updates on when we are going back. The last time she was out she noticed me pushing on my side. I informed her that I was dripping again. She told me to come back with her. We went to the locker room. I met some of her coworkers, and they couldn't believe how much we look and sound alike. Anyway, she took me into the bathroom, and I showed her the drain. Well, she told me that it was more than halfway out and that she was just going to take it out! Yikes! But when she took it out, I didn't feel a thing. She was right, I didn't know how it even stayed in there. How embarrassing would that have been if my drain would have fallen out while I was walking! While we were in the bathroom, the nurse was looking for me since it was time for me to prepare. It is really nice knowing people at the surgicenter—a definite feeling of comfort. Kathy got me all pre-opped, and this time, I didn't wear any jewelry. The anesthesiologist came in and got my hand. It is so nice that they can numb you prior to the IV going in. Kathy wrote yes on the left "breast" and on my right arm. Dr. Warren came in and signed on it as well. Mom came back, and then it was time for me to go. They asked me if I wanted to walk there, but I informed them that I was really blind, without my glasses, I can't see too much. So I got the royalty treatment, and they rolled me in there. On the way, I found out that Dr. Warren's patient after me cancelled. I told her I did this because I wanted all of the attention on me. HA-HA! If you remember, last time, all of her patients cancelled due to illness or not following fasting directions. It is cold like before and we are in the same room. I was knocked out much quicker this time because I don't remember anything. In fact, I don't even remember where I woke up—in the operating room or the recovery room. Wow, they gave me some powerful stuff that time. Anyway, the drain is in again, and they took the IV out. It was about one in the afternoon, and I was able to get dressed. While I was getting dressed, I noticed that my drain is not keeping suction. I let the nurse know, and she called Dr. Warren. In the meantime, Brenda got another ball to make sure that it is not that. We thought it was working, and then, pop went the suction again. The nurse told us that Dr. Warren told her to put more Bacitracin around the drain and surgical site to close up any air that may be getting in. We tried that, and so far so good. By the time I got home and walked into the house, the suction was gone again. I ended up calling Dr. Warren, and she called back and told me to try the Bacitracin again. If it doesn't hold, then I would have to come in on Monday, and we will take it out. It may be because I had the previous drain in for so long that the skin has widened and does not keep suction. I have not had to take any pain medication, but I am feeling a little tired. I reassured my mom that I will be fine and that she doesn't need to stay. I grabbed a bite to eat—my favorite meatloaf, and then I went to lie down. The boys came home and came back to check on me. I reassured them that I am doing okay but just tired. So, Bill took them out to play some kickball. I could hear them from the window and wanted to be out there so badly. I got a little shuteye, and then Zachary came back crying, saying that I was going to be mad at him because he took off the pedals of the flower outside. Then Buddy came back, telling him to leave me alone and that Daddy already told him that they will grow back! Isn't it funny how kids just need their mom for certain things?

Joanne came to check on me and told me to lie on my side and see if that helps with the suction. It did for a little while, but nothing was draining. I rested for the rest of the day. Bill, Joanne, and my mom were getting ready for the townwide yard sale tomorrow in Delaware City. I am glad that I am feeling so good. Dr. Warren said that I probably won't feel too much since she is taking something out, not putting something in.

Before I went to bed, I checked out the site. There was a yellowish piece of material over top of the stitches. I told Bill that they have that there so that grass will grow! Really, it is an antibiotic patch, but it reminded me of the stuff they put on the ground to make grass grow. With that said, I was off to bed.

Saturday, April 26, 2008

Bill had an early morning getting the stuff over for the yard sale. Then he got Zachary to his ball game at 9 a.m. Buddy and I took our time, and I was feeling good. No pain, just the drain with no suction. I headed over to the yard sale, and it felt okay to drive. But I take the back roads just in case. It was a very nice day to be outside. I didn't do much aside from sitting and talking, better than being at home because I know that I would try to do more than what I should because I felt so good.

While I was there I met Dave's mom's neighbor who was going through treatments for Breast Cancer. Bill & I spent a good period of time talking with her and her family and reassuring her that losing her hair would not be as bad as it she thinks (She was starting chemo the following week). I did add her to my list of great people that I have met along the way.

Later in the day, we packed up and got ready for Buddy's ball game at 4:30 p.m. It has gotten much colder and windy out since earlier, but it was nice to be there to watch the game. When we got home, I took a look at the site. Things were looking good. The tissue redness was going away already. My port site was more sore than where the expander was taken out. I am glad that both were taken out, but boy, was it easy to get blood drawn with the port in.

Sunday, April 27, 2008

It is my nephew's birthday today, and we went to the skating rink for a party. Since I didn't want to get on skates, we waited till Bill got off work. He would meet us there. What I was realizing was that the drain wasn't too bad when it kept the suction, but now that it doesn't, it sure does take up a lot of space. I ended up wearing a dark shirt and trying to cover it. Oh yeah, and taking a shower with it is for the birds.

The boys had fun, and while I was there, I ran into one of the nurses from the HGC. She remembered me and commented that my hair looked good. I think it so funny how so many people think that I have put the "frosted" spot in my hair. It also catches me off guard when total strangers come up and tell me that they love my haircut. If only they knew how I got it this way!

Monday, April 28, 2008

I called Dr. Warren's office first thing in the morning. The girls were surprised and wanted to know how I got the number. I informed them that

Dr. Warren gave it to me and told me to call. I had an appointment at 9:45 a.m. When I got there, she said she knew that it was just that I wanted to see her. She looked at the site and said that everything was closed and that it didn't look like there was any sign of fluid buildup. We thought that the drainage before was due to the overly irritated area from the expander. Another good reason to have had it removed. She cut the stitch that was holding the drain, and out it came. Gee, I didn't feel a thing. I must be getting used to it. She told me that she will see me next week to get the stitches out, and then after, that it will be about a month before I need to see her again. I may go through withdrawal.

I left there and headed off to Strasser's office to reschedule my CAT scan. Karen calls me her problem child, but was glad to hear that things are finally coming along. Dr. Strasser said he wanted to see me, so we went into a room. He looked at the site and said that we will wait one more week before doing the scan to make sure all healing continues. I talked with Karen again, and we set the appointment for 9 a.m. on Monday, right after I get my stitches out. The following week should be when I finally start my radiation. Later, Buddy had an appointment with Kym. She said that things are going well and that she doesn't need to see him for two months. She told me that I always surprise her. Buddy told her that I had surgery on Friday, and she couldn't believe that I was sitting there like I had nothing done. Hey, you gotta keep on movin'. Buddy's ball game was cancelled due to the rain, so we just hung out at home and got the house ready for the carpets to be cleaned. I tell you, some days Buddy can be the best helper. He took everything off his floor, and he even cleaned the bathroom. No questions asked. Now Zachary on the other hand still needs a little help, but I know that will come in time.

Tuesday, April 29, 2008

Kids were off to school, and the carpets were cleaned. Darla had made some nice spots on the carpet. I got a lot of calls out of the way and checked my e-mail. Later, I took a break and closed my eyes for a little bit. We had scouts later that night. We are going camping this weekend so we need to talk about what to bring. After scouts, the boys got ready for bed. I can't remember what I was doing, but I reached over near my "once breast," and it took me by surprise when I didn't feel anything there. I mean I am flat! I felt like I am half-man, half-woman, I remember dressing up as that one year for Halloween, but never did I think it would come true! See what cancer does to you. I am losing my boobs, getting hairier, what next? You know that I am just kidding with this! Just want to make sure that you are still smiling. But in all seriousness, I will say it does feel so weird not to feel anything over there.

Wednesday, April 30, 2008

Buddy had his first filling today at 11:10 a.m. He got picked up early today. While I was getting ready, I encountered my first lopsided situation. What do I wear? Can you really tell the difference? Should I stuff it? Here I am, thirty-seven years old, and I am stuffing my bra with a sock! It doesn't look too bad; it is not as full, but since the stitches are in, I don't want to press too hard against it. The girls at work couldn't tell and said I looked good. It was nice to see that Dr. H has written an update on me in the office for my patients to read. That meant a lot to me. I ran into some patients, and they were very excited to see me. I do miss it.

Buddy did great! He didn't even know that he got a needle but said that the numbness felt really weird. I had lunch with some of the girls and got caught up on their lives. It was nice.

Thursday, May 1, 2008

One of the steri-strips came off where the port was removed. The incision site looks like it is going to look better then when it was placed. The bruising is still there and a little sore but getting better. Buddy had his pre-op appointment today for his surgery on Tuesday. He did really good and actually answered the nurse when she asked him questions. I did have an embarrassing moment while we were there. We got on the subject with the nurse practitioner about my cancer and how Buddy is aware of surgeries and IVs since I just had one on Friday. Buddy then proceeds to tell the nurse that his mommy has a sock stuffed in her bra! (He overheard me telling the girls at work, that is how he knew.) We all laughed hysterically, and my face did get red. Kids will say the darndest things. I did tell him later that that is something that we don't have to tell people.

We went to pick up Zachary, and then Bill and I got our picture taken for the Christiana Care Focus publication about the study group that we are going to be a part of. So if any of you got that, look for the article around the end of the month.

We took the kids to Toys R Us. They got a toy, and we went home to play with them. My mom came over to see how everything went. By the way, she is doing fine. No injuries from her "fall." I got her to come into the bathroom so I could show her the site. When I told her to look, she asked me what I wanted her to look at. She has never looked at any of the other sites, but she did look at this one. There isn't much to see, just skin and stitches.

Friday, May 2, 2008

I continued to feel really good. Bruising was getting better, and there were no openings anywhere. I sat typing my update, knowing that I have to get ready for our overnight camping trip with the Cub Scouts at Killens Pond. Pray for a dry weekend.

My upcoming events will be suture removal and CAT scan, and I am going to have to go shopping for a prosthesis. It is going to be a while till I start with reconstruction again. So in the meantime, I will have to get something to make me look even. I can't be using socks all the time. I also have to remember that summer is coming, and we are planning a two-week vacation to Florida in July. I thought that I would have been done all treatment by now, but obviously I am not. Bill and I have discussed it and said we are not going to cancel it. It will actually be nice to get away for two weeks without having any doctor's visits. I will finish up radiation around June 18, and I will need the skin to heal. But I will also need to be extra careful while in the sun. It will be a tough summer. Also, I have to consider a swimsuit. I will again experience something new. I can't wait!

I appreciate all of your kind words and comments on how I have helped some of you in the way you look at things in life. Living is a good thing, and I plan on doing plenty of it. So until you hear from me again. Have a great day! Summer is right around the corner.

I Am Free!

S titch-free, that is!

Hey there, everyone! I hope all of you are doing well. For all of the mothers out there, I hope that you had a great Mother's Day!

My camping trip with the Cub Scouts was great. Thank you for all who prayed for dry weather because even though it looked pretty tempting, the rain held off for our events. It was a nice getaway for the kids and the adults. It also felt really good that I didn't have any drains hooked to me during that.

Sunday, May 4, 2008

It is Bill and I's twelfth anniversary. We weren't in Hawaii (where we honeymooned), but we were together during the day, and he had night work at night. As we say, we feel like we are newlyweds all the time. I can hear some of you now saying "Oh please!"

Monday, May 5, 2008

I had a busy day as usual, and Bill was able to accompany me even though he was just getting off of night work. We went to Dr. Warren's at eight in the morning. All was looking good, and she was ready to take out the stitches. Before doing so, Bill asked if he could watch. She said yes, and I told him it was okay as long as he doesn't ask to take them out himself. I don't know how many stitches I had, but they are all gone! I am stitch-free! She told me that she wants to see me back in the middle of my radiation, which will be in about three weeks. This is just to check how the skin is doing. Bill asked her a little about reconstruction, and she informed him that it won't be for a little while before we start to move forward. She said that my body has gone through quite a bit and will need some time to "calm down." When we do start, it will depend on what the tissue looks like and how much we will be able to expand. If we can't expand to match the other "breast," then we may have to take some fluid out of the other one or take some skin from my tummy or back to help the expansion. Okay, let's just wait to talk about that. I won't see Dr. Warren till May 27.

My next stop is to Dr. Strasser's. He continues to joke with me. Prior to coming in the room, he was saying, "I really don't want to see this patient who is in room three!" Yeah, it was me. He looked at the site and was happy to see that all of the stitches are out. But he wants to wait one more week prior to starting radiation. This way, we have one more week of complete healing just in case something is still open! No, we aren't nervous or anything! Bill went in the waiting area, and I was taken back to get the CAT scan redone. (It was nice of him to say that he was not charging me for this one since it wasn't my fault that we had to do more surgery. There are still some decent doctors out there who aren't just about the money). I laid on the table, and they brought back my mold. I was able to put my arm back further so they put air back into the mold. It allowed them to remold me. It was a little uncomfortable, but if this allows the radiation to get at a better angle, I will be strong. They also had to give me another tattoo since my arm position has changed. I have up to four tattoos now. I think I am getting addicted! Once they (there is a trainee in there today) got me positioned, they stepped out of the room and started the CAT scan. Oh my, my fingers were starting to get numb in this position. I hope they hurry up!

It was finally over. It wasn't long, but you know when you want something to move faster and it doesn't? I slowly put my arm down and got the feeling back in my fingers. They told me that I will come back next Monday, the twelfth, for some X-rays, and then I will start the radiation the next day, the thirteenth! They gave me my check-in card with my barcode on it and my time is 9:45 a.m. every day for twenty-eight days. I got dressed and saw Bill very relaxed in the waiting area.

We then picked up the "hoopty" from the garage and headed home. We took a nap, which Bill was excited to do because he knew he would be able to fall right to sleep knowing that I was next to him! Boy, do naps go by fast. We got up and went meet Buddy at his book fair. We also got all of his schoolwork that we will miss next week, picked up some juice and ice pops for his surgery tomorrow, picked up Zachary, and headed home again. The boys played outside for a while. We ate, and then it was time for Buddy to get ready for tomorrow. He didn't seem nervous at all, thank goodness.

Tuesday, May 6, 2008

We had to be at A.I. Hospital by 8:45 a.m. His surgery was scheduled for 10:05 a.m. We dropped Zachary off at school and headed north. Oh, how I do not miss driving into Wilmington to go to work (I worked in Wilmington when I was a Dental Assistant). We were stuck in some traffic, and Bill handled it so well! He didn't get road rage once; in fact, he kept smiling the whole way, sarcastically of course. We got there and signed in. Buddy played on the computer prior to being called back. Once called back, he got his vitals done and headed back to his "room" to get changed. There were so many kids in the preparation area. Busy day. He got settled in, and they gave him some medicine to relax. He was pretty relaxed prior to taking the medicine, but this made him even more so. His eyes started to get glossy, and he was squeezing his lip nervously. The doctors came to talk to us prior to surgery to explain what will go on—pre-, during, and post-. Then at about 10:20 a.m., they were ready to take him back. We gave him a kiss and told him we are proud of him and love him. He just smiled. I looked at Bill, and he said he could cry! We headed off to the waiting room for the next hour or so. It went by pretty quickly. Dr. Luft came out about 11:40 a.m. and said all went well. There was fluid in both ears. Buddy should notice an immediate difference with hearing! He gave us the post-op instructions and said they will be out for us shortly. We got the call to go back, and oh let me tell you how different it is when you see your child lying in the hospital bed! I felt a little nauseated seeing all of the tubes, not that there were many, but still. He had some blood on the corners of his mouth and around his nose holes. He was just "waking" up. He looked at me but then went back down. The nurse said not to be surprised if within the next fifteen minutes he would be complaining that he is hurting. At that point, we will give him some Morphine. She was right; about fifteen minutes later, he was saying how he hurt. The nurse went to give him Morphine, but the anesthesiologist didn't put the dosage. Well, you know how long it seems when you are waiting for an ambulance? That is how long it seemed before they could get in touch with the doctor. Buddy was crying. It hurt so bad, and it hurt us not being able to do anything. I got a little nauseated then too. Bill and I stayed calm, knowing it wasn't the nurses' fault. The Dr. finally called back, and they got him medicated. He went back to sleep for a little. We were to stay in the recovery room for two hours just to make sure all was well prior to being sent home. When he was waking up again, the nurse offered him an icee, and he did drink it. It was a little after one in the afternoon when we were able to leave. Buddy didn't have that much color to begin with, but when we left, he didn't have any color. Poor thing. We, of course, took pictures along the way. You know me and my scrapbooking! He slept on the way home and pretty much the rest of the day. Uncle John stopped by with some goodies for Buddy, and then later that night, mom-mom stopped by with an Icee, balloon, and a Webkinz® pet, which he named Softback. My mom loved every minute of how lovable Buddy was toward her. He didn't want her to leave his side. Mom doesn't get to see that side of him too often. Bill and I were very proud of him during all of this.

You know how I say that things happen for a reason? Well the next couple of days were doctor-free for me. I could focus strictly on Buddy. It was nice to get things done and not think about cancer, doctor's visits, therapy, etc. I really felt like "me" and that I was a mom again. Bill didn't have to work so Buddy got a good amount of time with us. Of course, I think that he liked Daddy a little more because every time I got around him, I would bring out the homework. I don't think that I would be able to home-school. Kudos to anyone who does that.

Saturday, May 10, 2008

Happy birthday, John! Buddy started to feel a little better, and we ventured to a dog parade in Delaware City. We—Joanne, Jessica, Jaylyn, Diva, Brenda, Dudley, Buddy, Zachary, Darla, and myself—were dressed up in camo gear and had the wagon decorated. We won second place for most original and won $50! Buddy ate a soft pretzel while we were there, which is good considering he has been living on icees. His belly did get a little upset, but he was glad to be out. I saw some more friends whom I haven't seen in a while. It is nice to hear that you look good. I really feel good and want it to stay that way. Later on, I had a baby shower to attend. A friend of mine adopted a baby boy, Paul, from Guatemala. I am very happy for them, and Paul is adorable! I again saw a friend whom I have not seen in about a year. She had heard about what I have been going through and was happy to see me. After that, I headed home, and Buddy's game was cancelled. We were going to take him over there to watch but not play. His energy is not up to speed just yet. So, I got ready for a surprise get-together for John at Kelly's in Port Penn. Mom stayed with the kids, and they did great! It was nice to get out and socialize. I came home, and Mom had most of the kids (Jessica and Jaylyn had spent the night) to sleep. Of course, by morning, they were all in my room in the bed and on the floor. Bill was on night work.

Earlier today, when we were getting ready for the parade, Mom was asking how everything was healing up. I said it has been great, and there was no more leaking. Well, I spoke too soon! When we were getting ready to leave, I noticed that my shirt felt wet, and when I lifted it up to take a peak, my dressing was wet. I had been leaking! Everybody left, and I went back to change my shirt and dressing real quick. When I did that, I looked at the site, and oh no, I saw another protein bubble like before. I gently wiped off the area, and POP, there goes a gusher again. I didn't panic, and I cleaned everything up. It was a beautiful circle. No redness, no bleeding, just a perfect circle. I got more dressing, taped it up, changed my shirt, and headed on out. I didn't have time to worry about it. I went on with my activities, and when I came home to get ready for the baby shower, I took a peek, and I didn't see the hole anymore. It looked like it was closing up. I didn't pull on it too much because I didn't want to disturb it. I will tell you though that the side close to my underarm had some extra skin. I had to clean it like heavy people have to clean their folds. It was nasty. I mean, I keep it clean, but yuck! I hesitated to tell my mom because I knew that she would worry. But after I saw that it looked like it was closing, I told her. I think it just wanted one more hoorah!

Sunday, May 11, 2008

Happy Mothers' Day! We had cake for breakfast, Joanne's favorite. We (Joanne and I) ended up not doing too much. We were tired and had the perfect excuse not to do anything. Bill was coming off of night work so we went down to Joanne's and just vegged out. Later that night, we were going to our friends' Scott and Stacey for a cookout. It was nice not having to cook; I just needed to bring my famous deviled eggs. They played some wiffle ball, I was just not ready to be that active, and then when it started to rain, we went inside to play some game on play station with a guitar, drums, and a microphone. It was a lot of fun and was great seeing all of us having a good time. As I was sitting there drumming, I noticed that my bra, left side of course, felt a little pushed in, so I slowly went into her dining room to readjust. To my surprise, I forgot to put a sock in it! Oops, good thing I was not wearing a form-fitting shirt. I think it is time to go shopping for my prosthesis.

I entered my mom in a contest for Mother's Day at "Forget Me Not" florist. She won third place and got a beautiful flower arrangement. It was a nice surprise for her. I love you, Mom!

Monday, May 12, 2008

Happy first anniversary, Brenda and Dave! Buddy is back to school and feeling good. I am sure that he will be pretty tired after he comes home. I had my appointment to get my X-rays done prior to radiation. It was done in the same room as where I would get the radiation. I got on my pretty gown and waited to be called. Once I got in there, they positioned me in my mold, moved me around some, and told me that they were going to be taking some X-rays and that I need to stay still. They were not too talkative, and they didn't say what they are doing. You know me, I want to know everything that they are doing. I am going to have twenty-eight days with these girls? It is going to be a long twenty-eight days. As I lay on the table, I looked up and found out that they have a pretty scenery in the ceiling light, like in the CAT scan room. The music was playing, and they left the room. It was very open in there so there was no fear. To my right were a couple of computer screens. I was almost straining my eyes to read them, but I didn't understand what any of it means. I heard some beeps, and the machine was moving some. The nurse came in and re-adjusted me and left the room again. At this point, my hand started to feel uncomfortable, and the mold wasn't the softest thing for your head. When the nurse came in again, I asked her if I could just lift my head and put it right back down. She tells me, "No, sorry, you have to keep still. You will be done shortly." I guess it was shortly, and then they all came in. There were three of them. They told me that I could get up. Oh, how stiff you get trying to be still and being so tense. They told me that they will see me tomorrow for my first treatment. I asked if Bill can come back tomorrow to see the room and to take some pictures, and they told me yes. I got dressed, and then I went to see Strasser. I will see him every Monday just to have him check and see how the skin is doing. He sat and chatted with me for a little. I showed him the site, and he was not too concerned with the opening. It looked pretty small and looked like it was closing. I was done for the day, and it was eleven thirty in the morning.

I came back home, made my phone calls to update my family. This is when I get disgusted, not with my family, but with my insurance company. Remember when I told you that I got a check for $72.10 for my wig? Well if I didn't, then I just did. I sent that back, and they resubmitted it saying that it should have gone to Pennsylvania instead of New Jersey since that is where the boutique was. Well, to make a long story short, I called them again; and they informed me that that is what I will be getting back. I do have a $250 deductible and a co-pay which leaves $72.10 that they covered. The lady told me that my policy states that I have a $750 lifetime coverage for wigs after my deductible and co-pay are reached. Did anyone tell me that when I called two times prior to purchasing it? They have it in their record that both times they reviewed it with me. Don't you think that as anal as I am about details, I would have asked them what my deductible and copay is prior to purchasing the wig? Anyway, the money is gone, and my point of being agitated is that you try and check all of your information and you still can't get a correct answer from people. I have been dealing with this since December! Oh, but if you owe them money, you better get it to them within two days. Okay, I need to stop, I have vented enough. My blood pressure is rising, and I can't sweat the small stuff.

I picked up Zachary, and wow, what a miserable, rainy day. I got home, and Bill was running late for work. Buddy was having trouble with his homework. Jessica was trying to get the fax to work since she forgot her homework. The TV downstairs was not working, and I was trying to start dinner during all of this. I felt myself getting very freaky and wondered if it is a full moon or if this would be my time of the month. (Luckily I still have not had a menstrual period, but I do think that once a month, the hormones still go crazy!) All finally calmed down, and I felt drained, so off to bed we went.

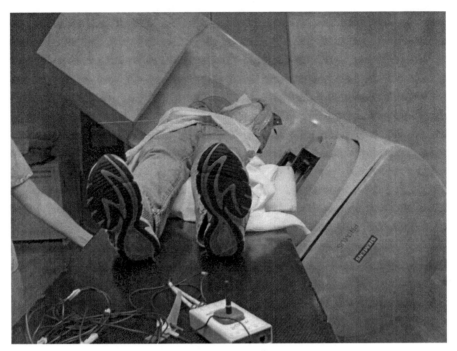

Photo session prior to my radiation treatment

Tuesday, May 13, 2008

This was my mom-mom's lucky number. This was the day of my first radiation treatment and the start of, let's see, phase three of my treatment, which sounds good. Bill went with me. Again it was at 9:45 a.m. We dropped Buddy and then Zachary off at school. Our plans were to go to Lowe's and the bank prior to that, but we sat and talked with Zach's teacher for a little while. I don't know why, but the hormones were raging again! Bill said that we needed to go and I, that quickly, forgot that we were going to go to those places prior to going to the doctor. I angrily said that we weren't going to have time to go there. Bill got a little disgusted, and then I said, "Fine, then let's go!" He of course became stubborn as well, and we walked to the car and didn't speak the whole way to the HGC. Once we got there, we were forty minutes early. He turned off the car, put down the windows, laid his seat back, and closed his eyes. I was totally wrong and just went crazy in my moodiness. It was time to go in, and we both had some time to relax ourselves. He asked if I was nervous for today, but really I was not. What I was not looking forward to is becoming tired later on in the treatment. I am just getting used to feeling like myself again.

I forgot my card, but the receptionist checked me in. I got called back and got changed. I realized that I am going to see the same people each day during my radiation. I have met a lady who is going through some lung cancer. They called me back, and my photographer came back with me. The nurses were more talkative today, and they were explaining to Bill what they were doing. Why didn't they do that with me? He got some pictures, and they positioned me. They told me that they have to get a couple more X-rays, and then they will start the radiation. The X-rays weren't bad, but my fingers were starting to fall asleep. She came in, readjusted the machine, and walked out again. She then came in and attached something to me and said that a total of three different areas will be getting radiation. She left the room, and here we go. All I could hear was the fans from the machine running. Then a beep went on. It stopped, and a couple seconds later, it sounded again. The nurse came in, moved the little sensor, and left again. Two more times of the beeping and then she came in again and said that this was the last time and then I would be done. Thank goodness because my fingers were tingling. I heard the beeps two more times, and we were done. Dr. Strasser's nurse was on vacation last week, but she came in to say hello to me and that she was glad to hear that we were finally starting treatment. Everyone is so thoughtful. I got changed, and I was done for the day. It was 10:40 a.m. We headed home. I started some house cleaning, and Bill went to lie down (night work tonight). I called my physical therapist to set up some appointments so I can get started with that again. We wanted to wait for some healing and keep some appointments available for during radiation. I also think that it will help with my fingers falling asleep when I have my arm somewhat above my head.

So here I am, giving you my update, and I am happy to say that I am feeling good, minus the raging moments. But that happens in everyday life. I hope that my radiation treatments go smoothly, and I just ask that you pray that they will. I don't need any more excitement, but if something does happen, I won't be surprised. I am happy that I am healthy enough to care for my Budman, and that he is doing good. I wish all of you a great week and hope that you get to spend some time with your family. Until next time, ADIOS!

I had taken a break in writing an update, and this is what I sent to everyone:

—

I just wanted to give you a very short hello. I am doing okay, feeling tired, but all in all, I am doing well. I have been busy, and I will be filling you in on all of my events, so be prepared. It will probably be a two-part update, but you don't want to miss it. So, any of you were wondering where I have been and if I am doing okay? Well, all is good, and I hope to get you updated next week.

We have our Relay for Life this weekend, and I am looking forward to a memorable and fun time. Also, my brother-in law-has finally come home from Iraq after twelve months! We are so happy for his safe return.

Here I Go!

Wednesday, May 14 and Thursday, May, 15, 2008

It was radiation at 9:45 a.m. The routine is quick to remember—scan your card, call me back, get changed (hope that there are pink gowns, I'll explain later), wait to be called, get radiated (six to ten minutes), get changed, and wait till the next day.

Friday, May 16, 2008

Happy Birthday Jessica!

After my radiation, I picked up a cake for my niece Jessica and went to her school for lunch. She was happy to see me, and the kids loved the cake. It was a pretty rainy day, but that made some sunshine for her! This is one of those times when not working is a good thing.

Saturday, May 17, 2008

Happy anniversary, Scott and Denise!

My first break from radiation. No signs or symptoms yet. Both boys had a game today. My mom took Zachary home, and Buddy and I went to Lums Pond for a campout with the Cub Scouts. This is the official crossing-over to becoming a Bear. The forecast said there would be severe thunderstorms, and Buddy said he didn't want to stay, but I had everything just in case. And being prepared paid off because once he got there, he changed his mind. Our luck was with us because it rained after we got in our tents to go to bed. It was a fun time, and I am glad that we stayed.

Sunday, May 18, 2008

Happy birthday, Jaylyn!

—

Joanne had a family birthday party for both of the girls today. It was a nice sunny day, and everyone enjoyed themselves. This day also ended in rain, but there was a short downpour, and then the sun was back out. The flowers and grasses love this.

Monday, May 19, 2008

This was doctor day. I received my radiation, and since it is Monday, I will see Dr. Strasser so he can check my skin and see if I am having any symptoms. I can't report of any; I am still very slightly draining in that one opening, but there's nothing to be alarmed about. I had some time before my next appointment, so I headed into Simply You at the HGC to check on some prostheses. If you recall, when I went in there for my wig, I just didn't feel that helpful feeling from the ladies. Well, the same thing happened again. I asked a question about the prostheses, and one of them said, "We have different kinds and sizes. What size are you? First you need to get a bra that fits you. We do have some prostheses that have been donated to us that might work." That was pretty much it. She didn't ask if I would like her to measure me or to see if I wanted to try on any bras/prostheses. Nothing! I asked her if I had to give her my name for the donated ones, and she said no and to just come back when I am ready. Ah, I think that was why I came in! I just can't connect with them, so I left.

I was off to see my gynecologist. She hasn't seen me since she sent me for the ultrasound in the beginning of this journey. I filled her in on ALL of my happenings, and she was glad to hear that she did not just blow it off to be a cyst. I am too! She checked all areas. What a joy. Then she looked at the "lumpy" flat breast. She was feeling around and stated that I have so much scar tissue on that side.

"Is that bad?"

"Not bad, it's just that you can feel it when I am checking for any other unusual spots."

She asked about the menstrual period and our form of birth control. She discussed a vasectomy for Bill (he wasn't there, or else I know that he would be cringing). Since I am no longer able to take birth control pills, we need to look at other forms of BC, and that one is the best preventative, unless you are Elaine and you are that one in how many to whom it can still happen! Anyway, we had discussed this after surgery anyway. Now it is time for Bill to go under the knife. Snip snip! I don't need to go back for another year unless the results come back abnormal.

Later in the day, I picked Buddy up for his post-op with Dr. Luft. We waited for close to an hour, but he said that all looked good. I was able to look in his ear at one of the tubes. How wild, it is green and so small. There are no precautions and no earplugs that are needed for swimming and bathing. He can't dive in five feet of water due to the pressure, but we are not at that point yet. He will see us back in November, and he will recheck him. He did not feel the need to retest his hearing as he knows that Buddy can hear better with the amount of fluid that had been removed. Don't I feel like a bad mother. How long had this gone on? Oh well, he is better now!

Tuesday, May 20, 2008

I had my sixth radiation treatment, and after every fifth treatment, they put this "bolus" material over my skin so that the radiation gets closer to my skin! Basically, this is what can make my skin turn red, gee thanks! It is only there for two of the positions. It feels like those sticky fingers that the kids get and throw on the wall, but it is thicker! It is funny, the position that I am in during my radiation enables me to see the computer screens, which is kind of nice. This way, I know that they have the right person because my picture comes up. On the other screen is where you see that the radiation is on. I would check to see that the same numbers come up. I am not really sure what the numbers mean, but I checked to see that they are the same each time. The first one was 111, then 68. Then the machine moved to the underneath, and it was 30, then 80. The machine moved again, but it was blocking the screens, so I couldn't see those two numbers. Oh well, by this time I knew it was for me.

I went to the mall to pick up a gift for my mom's birthday. Bill called to see if I wanted to meet him for lunch. We went to Bertucci's and had a nice lunch together. You gotta love the gift cards!

Later that night, since Buddy's game was cancelled due to rain, I took the boys shopping for birthday gifts for their dad. Zachary wanted to get Bill a cup, not sure what kind, but ended up getting him a pair of shorts (yes, I kind of helped). Buddy had said he wanted to get him a pair of chill pants (PJ pants), so I let him pick them out, and boy are they loud! They have the Simpsons all over them, and they are pretty bright. You gotta love it. When it is from your kids, you just don't care. Once Buddy started shopping, he couldn't stop. He also picked out a Phillies shirt, a pair of shorts, and a tank top. He said, "Gosh, mom, once you start looking at things, it is easy to shop for daddy!"

Wednesday, May 21, 2008

Happy birthday, Bill!

I got my radiation, picked up my boobie buddy Kathy, and we headed down to the Pink Ribbon Boutique to buy myself a boob! Not many of you can say that! The shop is in Smyrna and is owned by a survivor. It is small but quaint, and Terry was extremely helpful. We told her what I needed, and I didn't realize how many different prosthetics you can choose from. She showed me different sizes, shapes, and colors. There are ones that mold to your skin, some are more concave. Some have a "gel" pad that takes the heat off in the summer, and some are for swimming! Man, this is going to take a while. I started trying on different bras, and we placed different "forms" in. She did all kinds of measuring, and I explained what we were looking for. I didn't realize how involved she would be, but I am glad that we went there. Some bras really made me look lopsided, others just weren't comfortable. We finally found two bras that I liked and that felt comfortable wearing. The form that we chose was a "Swimform." This prosthesis is not as full in the back (near my skin), and it is meant for swimming. Since it is the summer time, and we will be doing a lot of swimming, I didn't want to get one that I would have to worry about it breaking down from the chlorine. It is less expensive, and it will also be able to be used during my re-expansion (if that happens) since there is room. I also had to get a new bathing suit since the ones that I have won't accommodate my "boob." You know how cheap I am, so seeing the price tag of $85 was pretty tough for me. But you gotta do what you gotta do. I got dressed and looked at some hats. Since I am going to have to be careful in the sun, I picked up a big-brimmed hat, which does look pretty cute. It shades a good bit of the upper part of my body. Okay, we better get the total. I didn't even worry about insurance because I may have my deductibles to meet again. So here it goes, $365. That is for two bras, one hat, a bathing suit, and the prosthesis. I got lucky because the other prosthesis cost around $300 alone. She has some that have been donated back that may be my size. She gave me one but thought it might be too big. My mom and dad had given me some money for this, so when I was finished, I called Mom up and told her she had just bought me a "boob"!

We were in there for a little over two hours! We decided to go get a bite to eat. You know that show Diners, Drive-ins, and Dives? Well we found a Dive, the Smyrna Diner. My friend has talked about this place, and you know how diners are usually really good? Well, the food wasn't bad, but the atmosphere was not the best. Poor Kathy, her bowels were a little messed up from her treatments, so she HAD to experience the bathroom more than once. I will have to say though that they are building a new diner, and I think that the upkeep of the place has gone downhill due to that. We ate our meal and headed home. We had another memorable day, and I am glad to say that the socks can go back on my feet and not on my chest!

Thursday, May 22, 2008

Happy birthday, Mom!

Can you believe all of the celebrations this month? The teachers at Zachary's school knew that I was going shopping for the "boob" yesterday, so I told them that I would bring in show-and-tell for them today. Don't worry; I made sure that none of the kids were around while I did this. I took in the donated one since that one looked more "real." The girls were amazed and didn't realize that is what it looked like. They were glad that I shared the information with them. Hey, I don't mind telling people; if you don't ask, you'll never know. Off to radiation I went!

We planned on going to Chincoteague this weekend, and we will celebrate all of the birthdays with cake down there. Can you believe that Memorial Day weekend is this weekend?

Friday, May 23, 2008

Radiation was at 9:45 a.m. They informed me that the machine that I am on is being transferred to another site and that they are getting a new one. This meant that I had to be moved to another room because the new one won't be ready until July! They only have a 7 a.m. and a 4 p.m. slot to choose from. Well, that's not going to work, so they said they will try and find something else. Oh darn, I was getting used to the 9:45 a.m. slot, and of course, I have met some nice people during that time. You know me, it is not hard for me to meet or talk to people.

I headed off to therapy, and they were all happy to see me. They love the hair. When Lisa examined me, she noted that I was pretty tight, but she doesn't want to push on the skin too much during my radiation. She would like to see me every other week just to loosen me up a little bit. After radiation, she will work a little "harder" on the site. She wants me to continue with the stretching, and we will keep a watch on lymphodema.

Buddy had a half-day of school and we picked Zachary up early. We headed down to Chincoteague for the weekend. My parents are already down there. We will also beat the traffic. I am looking forward to the weekend. Our whole family is going to be down there—kids, dogs, all of us. Joanne and Brenda hit some nice traffic and didn't get down till later in the evening. But we are all together, and that is what matters.

Saturday, May 24 and Sunday, May 25, 2008

We had some great time together and lots of food, of course. We went to the beach and the pool. It was pretty cold, but it didn't bother the kids any. We had our bonfires and plenty of S'mores! I also got to try my new bathing suit. It looks pretty nice, considering . . . My only problem is that it is a one-piece, and not that I am bikini material, but the tankinis give me more air. It didn't matter this weekend since it was pretty chilly.

We headed home on Sunday. Bill has to work overtime on Monday. This way, we can beat the traffic again. We all had a great time and look forward to the next time.

Monday, May 26, 2008

I hope that everyone had a great Memorial Day! The boys went swimming at our neighbors', and we just had a relaxing day. Bill had to work, but when it is on a holiday, the pay is good; and it is helping out right now.

Tuesday, May 27, 2008

I guess I had such a great weekend that I overlooked a doctor's appointment that I was supposed to have with Dr. Warren! I went to my radiation appointment, and they told me that my new time would be 1:45 p.m., and it would start next week. Dr. Strasser is out this week, so I saw one of his colleagues. Nothing new to report, and all looks good. I have noticed that the prosthesis that I have seems to "sag." (I think it is because it is concave and not up against my skin.) I feel like I am adjusting it a lot. Here I go again, feeling like a man, adjusting myself all the time. But mine is up top not down there.

So I stopped by Simply You to see if they had any donated prostheses that would fit me since I had my bra. The lady went to get one, and when she saw my bra, she said, "Where did you get that one, it looks like one of ours?"

I told her where I got it, and she said, "That is a cute place down there, isn't it?" She gave me a couple of other bras to try, and she left the room! She eventually asked how I was doing, and I asked her if she would come and check the "balance." She did some measuring and said it looked good. What a difference in customer—oh heck, I can't think of the word—you know, where they are helping you. Anyway, the prosthesis was a nice fit, and it is one that will mold to my skin when I wear it. I also got another bra that is pretty comfortable.

When I got home is when I realized that I had missed Dr. Warren's appointment. I decided that I will just go there tomorrow and apologize and get another appointment.

Wednesday, May 28, Thursday, May 29, and Friday, May 30, 2008

Not too much happened, just the radiation. I did go to Warren's and apologized for my forgetfulness. While I was rescheduling, Dr. Warren came out, and I apologized to her. She said "Don't worry about it, I am just glad that you are okay. When you didn't show up, I thought that you were sick from the radiation, so I am glad that it is not that." So I will see her on June 9.

We did have a picnic for Zachary's class at Banning Park on the twenty-ninth, and then I had two of his friends stay the night since their parents couldn't attend. It was easier and helpful to them for me to just take them with me. Call me crazy, but they were great, and everyone had a good time.

As far as symptoms, I still have no redness, but I am noticing that in the afternoon, once I sit down, I am done. I need to take a little nap. It is different than with chemo because with chemo, you feel sick, and you have to lie down. With radiation, I feel fine. I just feel lazy/tired, and that is hard for me since I like to be busy. I do listen to my body though and take a nap. After that, I feel better. Not one hundred percent fine but better. I also have noticed my throat hurting when I swallow solid foods. I remember one of the ladies stating that her throat was bothering her, but I didn't think that would happen to me because she is being treated for lung cancer. As I am becoming more aware of it, I mentioned it to Karen, Dr. Strasser's nurse. She stated that yes, it can happen since they are doing the chest wall and clavicle area but that it should only be on the side that is being treated, and it is. If it gets too painful, there is a medication that they can give me that will coat the throat, but I will hold off for right now. I am just learning to take a bite, and instead of swallowing once, it may take me four times to swallow. It is a tricky technique. You should try it sometime. It definitely will take you longer to eat. I am already a slow eater, so watch out if you eat with me now.

Saturday, May 31, 2008

Break from radiation for two days. We went to Buddy's game and then headed to the Monster Mile races in Dover with the Cub Scouts. It was again calling for some heavy winds and rain, but we attempted it. We got there, went to the kids' zone, got a snack, attempted to see some of the practice runs, and then it started to rain. They stopped the racing. We did some souvenir-shopping, and they started the racing again. But then it started raining again, and this time it did not stop. We headed back to the car, and we were drenched. We were prepared again. I had a change of clothes for the kids. We headed home and watched the updates on the TV, and I took a nap. We saw that they were going to start the races again, and the boys wanted to go back down. So we got in the car and headed back down. By this time, it was close to five thirty in the afternoon. The race had already started, but we all enjoyed ourselves. It ended up being a nice day/night. We look forward to going back in September, on a Saturday of course. I don't think we are ready for the Sunday crowd.

Welcome To Summer!

I hope that you are enjoying the official summer, considering it has only been a day! I have waited a little longer than I wanted for the update, but what are you going to do? Anyway, I hope that you all have some time to spend with your family and get away for a day or two. You deserve it and need to enjoy it!

Monday, June 2, 2008

I went to radiation, and they informed me that the machine is not being removed for another week or so! Yeah, I don't have to change my times. I did my normal routine for radiation, and then I saw Dr. Strasser. He didn't see too much redness, and I was not having any discomfort with anything. He informed me of the medications that he can give me if the throat becomes a bigger problem, but I am still okay for now. I will see him next week.

We—Zachary and I—went over to his pediatrician's office. Zachary was due to get some shots before he can go to kindergarten. Of course, Buddy informed him of the shots prior to our leaving. So this was all that he was thinking about. Once we got in the room and she came back in to give the needles, he went in the corner. I had to hold him down. Not a good thing, but the needles were so quick that it took longer for the tears to start flowing than it did for the needles to be put in. He got his Tweety Bird Band-aids and a sticker and we were on our way. Now, we just have to wait until August for his first day of school. He seems so ready. I keep him home from preschool today, and he just keeps on saying, "Mommy, I can't go to school because

I just got shots, right?" The rest of day, he was proud to show everyone his Band-aids and told them where they were from.

Tuesday, June 3, 2008

I did my radiation and then headed off to therapy. Again, it was a short session because she didn't want to irritate the skin. But she did some stretching on the arm range of motion. I told her I put on my watch today, and it felt tighter. She measured me again, but all looked okay. She said there was still a little swelling but not enough to be worried about. Thank goodness.

There was an Auxiliary meeting tonight, but I felt too tired to go. So we got our pajamas on and relaxed.

Radiation versus chemotherapy. Here is the difference between the two. During chemo, you feel sick and don't want to move or do anything. Radiation, on the other hand, doesn't make you feel sick, but you just don't have any energy. By the middle of the day, you are crashing and need a forty-five minute nap. Now, you all know that that is not my thing. I am on the go, but I do listen to my body, and I lie down for a nap. Once I do that, I feel better. It is hard though because you just feel lazy, and I am afraid of getting used to that.

Wednesday, June 4, 2008

Here goes a busy day! It was Buddy's last day of school! He took the bus, which is different because since my radiation, I have been taking him and then dropping Zach off and then heading to radiation. But today, he wanted to take the bus. Here is where that news is that I spoke about. I went to the bathroom, and of course, you know me, excuse the details, but I normally am wearing a panty shield, and today I wasn't. When I looked down, I thought to myself, *Did I pee* (you know, dark underwear) *or is that what I think it is*! Yep, it's back! I sat there and counted how long it has been. Well, I guess my "pregnancy" is over because it has been nine months. Oh joy, so happy for its return. I don't think I would have been disappointed if it never came back. I have noticed that the hot flashes have gone away slowly. I guess that was a sign.

It is weird though because even though my last chemo was on January 3, I feel like it stays in your body for this long. I say that because I notice my nails. There is a dark line that you can see in my nail bed. As the nails grow, that line comes closer to the top. I know that they said that is from the chemo. So I am slowly getting back to normal, and "it" is getting out of my body.

Anyway, I had my radiation, stopped by the mall to get a gift for Buddy's teacher (nothing like waiting till the last minute), picked him up McDonalds per his request. He said a lot of the kids are having their moms bring McDonalds for the last day of school picnic today. Whatever happened to the real picnic food?

I dropped by his school, and he had told me earlier that he wanted to stay at school today and not go to Uncle Dave's homecoming celebration. But he felt bad. I told him that Uncle Dave will understand if he is not there and that he can see him this weekend. Buddy enjoys school, and you know how that last day of school is. He had a movie, a picnic, and prizes. He was making sundaes with his Kindergarten reading buddy. So he understood that I wasn't able to stay for the picnic and would see him at home later that day. So, off to the welcome-home celebration for Dave. We all wore our blue shirts that had his name on it. It was at the New Castle National Guard center because it was supposed to rain, and Delaware City doesn't have a place to accommodate. Anyway, it was an emotional event. I did not think that I would get that emotional, but I did. It was great to hear that all one hundred forty-eight (I think) members of the one hundred fifty-three MP units returned home safely! My sister and Dave were even on Channel 3 news. I, of course helped out with that. I saw the newscaster and went up to her and asked if they were looking for a good story. I explained how they had gotten married right before Dave left and that now they can work on their honeymoon. So they got the reunion on camera and interviewed them! It was pretty cool! We went back to Brenda's for a celebration and watched the news. Once I got home, we had dinner, and then we headed off to our last Relay for Life meeting. I am hanging in there, while at Brenda's I got my rest time in. We got last-minute information and the T-shirts for our team members. On the way home, the boys were asking to see Uncle Dave, but because of the time, we just called up there for them to say hello to him. It is nice to hear that they missed him and are glad that he has returned home! Okay, I am ready for a good night's sleep—or not!

Thursday, June 5, 2008

Oh my gosh! Okay if you are a male you may want to skip this part. I feel like I need a blood transfusion. I had to wake up in the middle of the night and change. So you know that you are not getting a good night's sleep because you are so worried about leaking. Well, when I got up the next morning, I headed right for the shower. Is there something punctured inside of me? I have never bled this bad. As I am learning some of you experience this on a monthly basis. I am used to having my period for three to four days and changing the "T" every four to five hours. Well, not now. I got ready, went down to Joanne's, and darn if I didn't have to change again! Oh this isn't good. Joanne told me to plan my day accordingly and to be prepared. I went to my radiation and then headed right up to the oncologist's office where the nurse, Debbie, informed me that she has heard that when it comes back, it comes back with a vengeance! Well, for me it has. Needless to say, my day was pretty red. Both boys had a game that night, and I just don't feel like going anywhere during this time especially when the bathroom is a port a potty. UGH! I made it through, and now it is bed time. I have never done this but am told it is okay. I slept with a "T" and a "P" and still had to get up and change. Enough already! I am ready for this day to be over and hope that things slow down.

Friday, June 6 and Saturday, June 7, 2008

I went to radiation, and they told me that next week is when my room and time will change. It looks like they can get me in at 11:45 a.m. I have to say that the nurses/technicians are so nice in there. They are always asking how I am doing, and they never seem to be rushing you. It is nice to know that during this time that the people enjoy what they do, and it shows!

After radiation, I went home to get a bite to eat. Bill was packed for setting up the relay and told me to hang at home for a while and rest before heading down. So I did and got down there about one thirty in the afternoon. There was about five of us who set up the site. We went home, showered, and then headed back down for the night.

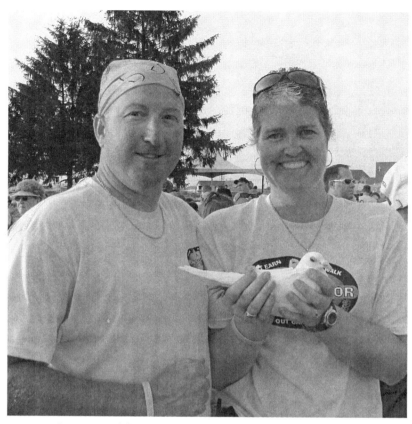

Survivor celebration at the Middletown Relay For Life

This is the event in a nutshell. IT WAS AWESOME AND EMOTIONAL! They had a survivor's dinner at six in the evening and then a survivor's lap at seven. But before the lap, they had all the survivors release doves! It was great. What was so special was that Bill and I released doves at our wedding! The funny thing is that my boobie buddy, Kathy, was so afraid of the dove. She is not a bird person, and the expressions on her face were hysterical. But after it was done, she expressed how great it was! We took our first lap, and my mom and Joanne (I found this out later) were pretty emotional during this. It was a proud moment for me! The night continued with everyone taking turns walking the laps with our flag. There were a lot of people there. We had thirty-five members on our team.

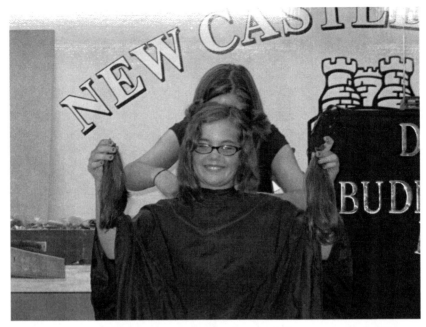

Jessica getting her hair cut to donate for wigs! I was so proud of her, she was leery of doing it but said that she wanted to do it for me!

My niece, Jessica, even cut her hair for Cuts for a Cure. She is such a sweet girl. She wanted to do it so bad but kept saying that she liked her long hair. I told her that she didn't have to do it, but she then said that she wanted to do it for me! My friend Lee gave her $20 for doing it. I was so proud of her. She always has a special place in my heart. Around nine in the evening, they held the luminaria ceremony, which is a time when we honor those who have won the battle, those who are fighting the battle, and those who have lost the battle. There were bags, which were decorated by family members. They had a candle inside, and they were lining the track. You stand next to a bag, which is usually one that you made up, and they say a few words. They announced different categories, i.e., "If you have a mother or father whom you are recognizing, please light your luminaria now." This goes on till they have covered all categories. Then a bagpiper plays while he is walking the track. It is a touching moment that you just cannot explain/ understand unless you have experienced it. I say that because my mom was so upset during that time because no one had made up a bag for me. I had tried to convince her that it was okay, and we can get it next year. Being that this is our first year, we didn't really understand how it worked or how touching it would be. Between this and the dove release, it is a close race on which one was more touching.

By the end of the night, the number of people got fewer and fewer. A good number of people that were going to stay didn't but for legitimate reasons. The kids hung in there and had a blast. A very special thank you to Joanne, Little Brenda, and Chrissi for hanging in there the whole night and making sure that our flag was on the track! The next morning, members had returned—thank you, Dawn and Jim—to help break down and walk. The weather was pretty hot and muggy on Saturday, but we hung in there and were happy that it didn't rain as it had in the past. There were more activities—a kids' walk—and then there were awards. I am very proud to say that our Team Survivor won "Rookie of the Year" (which was started because of us) since we raised $9300 for this event! Thank you to all who donated for this Relay for Life. I can't wait to do it next year!

Buddy is looking forward to next year too. He committed to going to his ball game on Friday night, so his coach picked him up. He unfortunately missed the dove release and some of the activities. As much as I wanted him to be there, it was important that he learns about commitment. Once he got there, he was okay. My mom and dad came back on Saturday and picked up the boys because they had a game at eleven thirty in the morning. After all the activities were done, and we were cleaned up, I headed home, and Bill headed over to the ball games. I left everything in the car, took a shower, and I think I fell asleep before my head hit the pillow! Oh yeah, and the menstrual period is done for this month!

Happy birthday, Brenda!

Sunday, June 8, 2008

We had a relaxing day, and the kids hung out at Joanne's pool. We went to the neighbors' for a cookout. Bill had to work, and then we called it a night.

Well, It Continues!

Monday, June 9, 2008

I had an appointment with Dr. Warren at 8:45 a.m. She was happy with the way the skin looked and how there was no more opening! She will see me after my radiation is complete, and then we will discuss what the next step is. I went to my radiation and saw Dr. Strasser. Oh yeah, I forgot to tell you about the pink robes. When we get changed for treatment, there are these cotton robes that we put on. The pink ones are the ones that are made for women. But they aren't always there. So, when the patients walk in, the first thing we ask each other is which room has the pink robes. If there aren't any, we have to wear these blue ones that—I swear—are made for men because even though you tie them, you still are flashing everybody your chest. Give me some beads! You have to find some laughter in everything you do, so that is what we joke about when we go to the dressing room.

I saw Dr. Strasser, and he was still happy with the skin color. He informed me that since my expander was out, he wants to add three more treatments right at the chest wall where the cancer was. I am okay with that—whatever it takes to rid of this for good.

Tuesday, June 10, 2008

Happy birthday, Cathy!

Bill went to radiation (my twentieth treatment) with me. We had our camera. We took more pictures of the room since the first ones didn't really turn out. He joked with Dr. Strasser and got his picture with Karen and I. They are so friendly and fun.

We stopped by my sister-in-law's to wish her a Happy Birthday. It was a nice visit. I am happy to say that the relationship with Bill and his sister has been very good for the past year. They had some rocky times, but it seems to have all worked out. I am happy to know that we can be around each other without any tension. As I have stated before, family is so important, and that is his family.

Later that night, Bill and I went to our first counseling session at the HGC. This was mainly an introduction session, and there were four other couples. I do have to say that I expected them to be younger. There was one other couple who is around our age. The rest of them are in their late forties, fifties, and sixties. One couple was going to have a hard time not because her breast cancer was not severe, but she had calcifications, and her treatment was radiation, and that was it. So the discussions didn't really pertain to her and her husband because the treatment she had was short. The other thing was that her husband has trouble hearing, and I don't think he heard anything that was being said. I hope that doesn't sound rude, but it is nice to have participation from everyone. They gave us a relaxation technique that we have to do over the next week. We'll see how that goes.

Wednesday, June 11, 2008

I started to get some itching and some bumps on my skin from radiation. After I got my treatment, we waited in the hallway for a lady whom I met who was about to ring the bell. This bell symbolizes the completion of your treatment. As we were waiting, Karen (Dr. Strasser's nurse) walked by and asked how I was doing. I told her I was okay and showed her the bumps. She told me not to pick them and that they are inflamed hair follicles. Interesting!! I also told her that I was a little itchy, and she told me not to scratch it but to pat it or push on the area. Scratching can irritate it. After she said that, Buddy chimed in and told her that I have been scratching it! She told me to put some hydrocortisone on it and see if that helps. My friend rang the bell, and we all cheered in celebration. My day will be coming soon enough.

Thursday, June 12, 2008

Happy birthday, Dad!

I went to radiation, and while I was changing, I noticed that my skin was starting to turn red. Also, when you touch the breast area and my flaps, they are not as flaccid as they used to be. They feel thick and don't move as easily. This also goes for my arm. When I lift it over my head or out to my side, I can definitely feel the tightness. I don't consider this to be too bad, considering that I was done over half of my treatment. After my radiation, they informed me that my time tomorrow will be at 11:45 a.m., and it will be in another room.

We went to my dad's for steak sandwiches, as per his request, for dinner and gave him his gifts. We are happy to say that dad has received his first cell phone. It is called the sixty-five-and-over phone! Even though he won't say it, I think he is happy to have one. A couple of years ago, we tricked him like we got him one, but to our surprise, he seemed a little disappointed that it was just a joke. Anyway, it was a great time for all of us to be together. Bill and I left to go to Zachary's ball game. The season is coming to an end.

Friday, June 13, 2008

The number thirteen must be my number like my mom-mom's was. That was her favorite number, and that has been the day that I started my radiation treatment. Now, it is the day when they are changing my times. Everyone knows how I am not good with changes. Well, the time change wasn't that bad, but the room change is an adjustment. When I had to get into my position, it just felt weird. Also, remember how I would look at the screen during my treatments? Well, the screen was on the other side of the room, so now I can't even look at that. My mind now has to just be on getting radiated. I don't think I realized how much looking at the screen took my mind off of what and why I was getting this done. Pretty weird, huh. The nurses were different, and that is a scary thing too. I was just wondering if they were lining me up the right way. The nurse did say I was perceptive because when I looked at the machine I noticed the pattern that the radiation came out of, didn't look like mine. She told me that they were resetting it, and then it will be the right one. She was surprised that I recognized that. You have to know your surroundings.

Happy Father's Day to all of the dads out there! The weekend was pretty uneventful, and I noticed more redness. The bumps have disappeared, some on their own, and some with a little help. I just couldn't resist.

Monday, June 16, 2008

I went to radiation and then saw Dr. Strasser. The nurse asked me if I have been putting anything on for the redness. When I told her no, she gave me some Aquaphor and told me to try that. When Dr. Strasser came in, he was joking, telling the nurse that she was spending way too much time with me and to get me on my way! He told me that if the itching gets too bad, he can give me a stronger ointment to use. He also informed me that the radiation is still working (burning) up to three weeks after my last treatment. I don't know if that is a good thing or not, considering that he noticed that my skin was looking redder. He was not concerned and will see me next week.

Tuesday, June 17, 2008

Happy birthday, Joanne!

It's the big 4-0 for her! We had a little cake and presents at my house. She doesn't know this but we are having a surprise party for her on Saturday at her house. She is going to be pretty surprised!

I headed off to radiation. I didn't wear my prosthesis today because my shoulder area was a little irritated. So I wore a black shirt to try and hide it. Well, you can't hide anything from Buddy because after treatment, when we were walking out, he looked at me and said, "Mom, why are you like this?" (He put one hand close to his chest and the other he puts out in front of him.) I laughed and told him why, but he already knew. I had to ask him to be quiet as I was trying to not make it that noticeable. Yeah, right. That made him have more fun with it. As you can read, I have continually kept the boys very involved with my whole process, and I feel that they can handle it better because I am not hiding things from them. Kids are stronger than we think.

Wednesday, June 18, 2008

It is getting harder and harder each day to take Zach to preschool/day care. Since the kids are off of school, he is realizing he is still going. Joanne has been taking him in the morning since my treatment time changed and the price of gas has gone up. Bill and I are going to talk about taking him out earlier than August 15, which we originally had planned. After my treatments are done, it will be easier because I will be home, but knowing that I have doctor's visits everyday is a little hectic with three kids.

My dad came over to watch Buddy and Jaylyn while Jessica and I went to a class at the HGC on organic versus natural versus whole foods. It was a brief overview on the differences. The biggest lesson that I got out of that class is that the cows for the organic milk are not treated with antibiotics for some illnesses. It is a personal preference on whether or not you want to go organic. I am sure there is more information that could have been given, but it was a half-an-hour class, and it was free.

I then went to my radiation and since the time changed, I didn't see anyone whom I saw before. There was never anyone in the dressing area except when I was done with my treatment. Jessica was intrigued by what I got done, and I think it helped her understand better too.

Later that night, we had our second counseling session. Mom and Joanne had the kids, and we left to be there fifteen minutes early like they asked. Well, we would have been there early if I remembered the right time. We left at five forty-five in the evening, thinking that the class would start at six thirty in the evening. Wrong, it started at six in the evening. It was storming that night, and when we got there, Bill (who wanted to be a storm chaser) wanted to watch the storm for a little bit. While he was sitting there, he said, "Are you sure that this starts at six thirty? Because I thought we were here earlier last time." Oh no, I have done it again. I looked at our folder, and sure enough, it started at six. We walked in fifteen minutes late, and they have started the session.

Our homework was to practice our relaxation techniques, and Bill and I didn't really have a stressful time that we had to use it. As soon as we sat down, the first question they asked us was: "How did your relaxation techniques go?" Don't we feel like the dunce? We were late, and we didn't do our homework! Anyway, the class was about communication with each other. We had to practice an exercise in class, but Bill and I just stared at each other and laughed. I hope we don't get kicked out of the class! We have more practice to do at home. We'll see how this one goes.

Thursday, June 19, 2008

When I went to radiation today, they put on the bolus material. But they told me that my upper chest, the position right above me, was done and that there were only two areas that they would be radiating. Yeah, it is getting closer to completion, only five more to go! I am hoping that since that one area is done, my throat will get back to normal. I still can't eat hard foods, and sometimes it hurts pretty bad but not enough that I want a prescription. This is only temporary, and let me tell you, it has not stopped me from eating like I had hoped. I didn't wear my prosthesis again due to some irritation, but I wore a button-down over the top of my shirt to mask the unevenness. After radiation, Zachary and I ran some errands, and then

I was off to get my first haircut! It was getting a little long over the ears and just needed some shaping up. I went to my friend Margie, and she cut out a lot of the curl in the back and shaped up the front. To my surprise, she even used a hairdryer on it. I didn't think it was long enough for that. Anyway, I really like it. I do miss the curl in the back, but I figured that I shouldn't get used to it since I know it is not going to be there forever. She gave me a courtesy cut and told me to put the money toward the Relay. Wow, I am collecting already for next year. Thank you so much, Margie!

When we left, Zachary kept asking me why I was getting it cut because I was going to look like a boy again. Kids, they say the darndest things!

Friday, June 20, 2008

I had Jaylyn and Buddy with me today. They were very good during my radiation, and again, the nurses were so accommodating with them. I again only did the two areas with the bolus, and when I left, I asked how many more just to double check. She explained that on Monday, I will be getting pictures, and they will be making a "pattern" around my scar tissue where the cancer was. They will line it up that way opposite my tattoos. She showed me on the screen the area; it was pretty interesting. After that, I will get three days of radiation, and then I will be complete! That puts it on a Thursday, so I am going to try and change the time since Bill is on night work, so he can take pictures of me ringing the completion bell. I will try to keep you posted on the time so that you can all keep an eye on the time wherever you are and shout hooray for me on that day! It was funny; in the room where I got changed, they had sheets of paper asking if you would like a celebration when you are complete, and if so, how would you like it done? How do you answer that question? How far would they go? I haven't filled one out because I don't know what to say. We headed home, and later in the day, I noticed a prickly feeling under my arm. I looked, and it was pretty brownish/red and a little tender. Yep, it does feel like bad sunburn. I put some ointment on it and hope that helps. It was a hard day because the kids were asking me to play some kickball, and I knew that I couldn't. Thank goodness, Aunt Doe Doe came to the rescue. Bill was working; otherwise, you know he would be running with them.

Saturday, June 21, 2008

Today was Joanne's surprise party. We were first taking my dad out for our annual Father's Day/birthday lunch with "his girls." We went over to New

Jersey at "The Orient." I did put on my prosthesis today due to the amount of public eye that I will be in contact with. We left at twelve forty-five in the afternoon and planned to be back by four thirty in the afternoon. Did you read that word *plan*? Because things don't always go as planned. Last year, we started another tradition to go to the "The Riverview Inn" for a drink out on the deck. Well, Joanne was ready to get her drink on. After one drink, Brenda asked for another, and Joanne followed her. At about four fifteen, I used the restroom and called Mom, who said that people were there and that they were starting to cook. I gave the signal that we needed to leave, and they finished their drinks. My family was concerned with me being in the sun, so they made sure that I was under the umbrella. The heat so far has not bothered the area. Anyway, we finally headed home, and Joanne had no clue. In fact, she wanted to stop to get another drink. Believe me, she is not an alchy, just enjoying the day. We pulled down the driveway, and she was so surprised. We pulled it off, and everyone had a great time. During the night, Bill brought the DVD that he made about the relay. He put in the first part about me and kind of the "path" that I have taken during my cancer. He used the song "Tough," which is such an appropriate song. It was then followed by all the footages from the relay. He did an awesome job, but the song and the DVD really touched Brenda so much that she couldn't watch it. Bill questioned himself that he didn't think that it was that sad, but I told him, "I don't think that it is sad because believe me, there are a lot of smiles on that thing." I think it is just the fact that you sit back and think, "Oh my gosh, my sister had cancer!" and it just brings the emotions back. I would love for you to see it, and Brenda, you know that we didn't mean to upset you. Know that I love you very much, and it is all going to be okay! Bill and I managed to get another night without any kids. How is this happening? Another good night's sleep, but I am noticing that it is not as comfortable sleeping on my left side, and when I do my stretches in bed, it feels really tight. But I know it is for my best interest to continue.

Sunday, June 22, 2008

Today, I went with my mom to visit my Aunt Sarah who has lymphoma. She is in her eighties and has been dealing with this for over a year. She has lost some weight since I last saw her but still looks good. I think that she really enjoyed the visit and asked that I don't wait as long next time. When you hear those comments, it always gets you thinking how you want to stop by every week and enjoy every minute that you have with her. I hope that

I will keep my word and get down there sooner than later. She is a strong woman and is enjoying her life as it is. She unfortunately has an inoperable tumor in her stomach, and she is not interested in doing any more chemo. In all honesty, I don't blame her, especially after seeing her and how happy and "healthy" she is. Please keep her in your prayers!

Later on in the day, I went to my boobie buddy's house because she was having a little get-together to thank all of the friends and family who supported and helped her during her treatments. It was a fun day, and the kids had a blast. Sounds like a great idea when I ever get finished with all my happenings.

Well, here we are at the beginning of the following week. I will see Dr. Strasser tomorrow, and I have my list of questions to ask him. I will keep you posted on the time of my last treatment so you can think of me and seriously yell HOORAY for me! I want to thank you again and apologize for the length of my updates, but as I have said before, it helps me get through what I have been through. I'll never know if you skim through it or actually read it. So my feelings aren't hurt either way. Anyway, I hope that you enjoy your day, and be happy with every breath you take. Don't forget, don't sweat the small stuff and try to look at the positive in anything that you do or that happens. Smile, someone is giving you a hug right now!

Hey there again,

You would think that I would have learned the first time, but I didn't. I just sat here and typed my past two days. And remember when it froze before and I lost it all? Well, I did it again, and I didn't save it as a draft. So here I am typing it all again. I won't even get into how I am really feeling right now. In fact, I am so angry, I have to get off of here and start tomorrow!

Get Ready To Shout Hooray!

Monday, June 23, 2008

I went in for my radiation, but I also got measured, drawn on, and I had an X-ray. I lay on the table, and they started with the measurements. Then they started drawing on me. Once they connected the dots with a pen that felt like a knife going along the areas that I have feeling, they attached this gadget to the machine that allows the radiation to come out closer to my skin. To give you a visual, it is a finger's length away and not an arm's length. I am a little intimidated by this. They asked me if I was ready. They walked out of the room, and about thirty seconds later, they came back in. Before I left, they explained what the boost was doing, but the only thing I heard was her saying that this is so the radiation can get deeper into the skin. They also told me to be careful in washing away the bright blue marker since that is what they are lining up with instead of the tattoos. Uh oh, this means no shower for three days! Just kidding, I'll be getting a bath and will be careful. I left and waited to see Dr. Strasser. Karen called me back, and I and my posse (Buddy and Jessica) came with me. She asked how I was doing, and I informed her of the sensitivity in my underarm. She took a peek and said it was peeling some, and it looked pretty dark. She said she is going to give me a sample of Xclare ointment to use for the next three days. She also gave me an Rx for silver sulfadiazine cream to use after that. This is the same cream that I used on the scab/wound in the beginning. FLASHBACK! Bring out the gauze and the tape again. I then asked her about my throat. It was feeling a little worse, and I am wondering if it is permanent and if there is something I can take with me on vacation in case it gets worse. She assured me that it will go away in about three weeks and that she'll give me another Rx for a medication that I will take four times a day to coat my esophagus. I also told her that my fatigue is a little more exaggerated. She called Dr. Strasser to come in, and HGC was having a T-shirt/hotdog giveaway to their employees. He told her that we were interrupting his hotdog. Well, when he came in, I told him to wipe the mustard off of his face! I was just kidding, but he grabbed a paper towel and wiped even though nothing was there. I got him that time. Anyway, back to business. He looked at the site and agreed that the meds that Karen talked about would be the best. He also stressed how important it is to be careful in the sun. The last thing I need is to get sunburn and a blister. Ouch! Well, it looks like I will be under the umbrella with my big-brimmed hat and having a T-shirt on while swimming. He doesn't have to see me for a month, and that is to check my skin. I asked him what he is going to do without seeing me. His response was: "I don't know, but what I do know is that I am glad we finally got started." He thought I was the longest he had to wait for a patient to start. Hey, what can I say, I like to make it memorable.

Later that day, we got lunch, went to Joanne's pool, and I was good in that I hung under the umbrella while I was outside. Bill played kickball with the kids, I started dinner, and then I went back in the pool for them. Afterwards, we all went outside and guess what we did. We tried to hula hoop. Main word here—*tried*. What has happened? I couldn't get it to go around more than two to times. The kids were having a blast watching us and showing us how easy it was for them. I even broke out in a sweat while trying. So guess what I suggest to you this time? Grab your little ones or big ones and get out there and be a kid again and hula hoop. You'll have a blast and a lot of laughs.

Tuesday, June 24, 2008

Joanne and I swapped kids. I took Jaylyn, and she took Zachary. Jessica went to work with Joanne today because she has a mole that needs to be checked out. Bill was home, so Buddy was staying here with a new friend who was visiting with his grandparents (our neighbors). I had therapy today, but like before, due to the burn, she couldn't do too much. She was going to stretch me as much as she could but would not touch the scar area at all. We have to wait three weeks for that. She suggested that I stretch as much as I can. She also remeasured me, and there was no swelling! I told

223

her that we will be going to Florida for two weeks, and she asked us if we are flying. Since we are and because of the length of time, she suggested that I learn how to bandage/wrap my arm in case of lymphodema. So I have an appointment next week. I would rather be prepared and hope that it doesn't happen. While I was there, she told me that I was brought up the other day. She said that during my whole process, I haven't complained once and that it is okay if I needed to. I told her that there really is no reason to complain. Even though I have had a rough time, it could have been worse, so I actually feel lucky. She told me that that is what makes me so inspiring and incredible. Even though I don't feel that I am doing anything special, it did make me feel good.

After that, I headed over to radiation. I used my little relaxation technique that I learned in my counseling class because I was feeling a little nervous about my first boost. They called me back. I was lucky enough to get a pink robe, and then they set me up. They lined me up with my outline and put the bolus—you know, the thing that makes me turn red—on me and asked me if I am ready. I told them that I am more nervous on this one because I feel like when it hits my skin, it is going to just sizzle. They reassured me that I will be fine and that the feeling is normal. They left the room, and I couldn't see the computer screen, so I didn't know the number. But it does sound longer than all of the others. It only did one shot and then they came back in the room again. They asked if it was as bad as I thought it would be, and I told them no.

When I left, I headed to Joanne's work to pick up Jessica so she doesn't have to stay there all day. I didn't have my prosthesis on, and I was feeling a little self-conscious even though I have masked it some with stripes. We then headed to Super G and picked up some things and a movie at this awesome machine they have where you can rent movies for $1. We have been doing this for the past week, and we have spent like $8 and seen eight movies. You can't even go to the theater for that price. We picked up Zachary and headed home.

Later that night, Mom came over to watch the boys because we had our third counseling class. We were going to do better this time since last week; we had a mess-up with the time. But we still didn't do our homework like we should have. This session was better; there was a little more discussion, and they discussed more techniques of communication. We had some homework that I believe we will be better at.

Wednesday, June 25, 2008

I headed to radiation, and Jessica accompanied me today. The set up was quick, and I asked if I could look at the screen. But it made my body crooked, so I just asked them what the number was. They told me 249. Yeah, that is longer than my others. Remember the first one was 111. I am not sure what they mean, but it makes me feel better that I know. I also asked them if the metal pattern on the gadget is strictly for me. They explained that it is and was made up when the original CAT scan was done. I asked what they do with it when I am done, and they told me that they melt it down and use it again. "Why, did you want to take it with you as a souvenir?"

"No, thanks, I can think of other things to have as a souvenir."

It is funny though. Missy, my nurse, first thought it looked like a flower, to which I said I had asked for a rose, but that was as close as they could get. She ended up saying that she changed her mind and that she thought it looked like a dog bone, not a flower. I think I like flower better. It surprises me on how many of the people that work there are aware that tomorrow is my last treatment and are expecting a loud ring. I am thinking that they know because I have practically talked to everyone there, but really I think it is because they really know what is going on with their patients. When I got home, I covered myself up with lotion and cream, used some bandage and tape, and "hung loose" in a different kind of way!

So for all of you, tomorrow is one of my big days! I changed my radiation time to 1:30 p.m. so that Bill will be able to be there for the bell-ringing. So tomorrow, which will be today for most of you when you read this, I would so appreciate it if you would yell out a loud HOORAY for me in celebration that my treatment is done. I know that I should be a little more excited, but I know that I still have somewhat of a road to go before completion. Don't get me wrong, I am ready for this chapter to end and get on with the next one. I will be anxiously waiting to hear the yells from all around, and thank you again for all of your support in my journey.

As I said before Bill, the kids, and myself will be going away from July 4 to 17. We are heading to Florida. This is the longest time for us to be away, but considering our year, it is going to be well-deserved. I am sure that I will update you prior to leaving, but until then, do me a favor and get out there and have some fun with the hula hoop!

I sent this out prior to leaving for vacation.

I just wanted to let you know that I am currently on vacation and totally enjoying this time. I know that I have not been able to e-mail you my emotional last day of treatment, but I can't wait to tell you all about it.

I will do my best to update you as soon as possible. I, of course, didn't want to leave you hanging as to how I did. I hope you all are enjoying your summer, and again, I cannot express the importance of spending time with your family! It is truly wonderful.

Also, on a sad note, I ask that you all pray for a good friend of mine who just lost her stepdaughter who was eighteen years old. It is going to be a trying time for her and her family, but the thoughts and prayers will do them good. Thank you!

I am going to try and give you an update while on vacation. The computer only allows me to type for twenty minutes, and I think all of you know that that won't be enough time for me. So for the next eleven days that I am in Florida, maybe I will have you updated.

Hooray Day!

Thursday, June 26, 2008

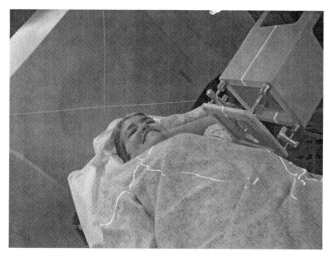

My last day of radiation

We—Bill, Buddy, Zachary, Jessica and I—went to my last and final radiation treatment! I am excited and not. I will explain. I am definitely excited that this is going to be my last treatment, but I would be more excited if this was the completion. I have a feeling that I have already told all of you this before. Oh well, I do know that I have a couple of surgeries to go through, but they shouldn't be that bad. I am excited that I will not have to go to the doctor EVERYDAY, but I will miss seeing the staff. Anyway, as you know, my appointment time was changed so that Bill could be there and then go straight to work. I usually get there early. Can you believe it? Me early? Well, Bill wanted to stop at Wawa and get a drink so we got there at one thirty in the afternoon. Once we got there and checked in, we sat for about twenty minutes, which only happens when Bill is with me. I went up to the desk and asked how much longer we had to wait because Bill was going to have to leave for work. She called to the back, and they told me to go back and get dressed. We all headed back, I get on my last pink gown, and then she called me back. Everyone headed back with me, and Bill took another picture. They got me set up and left the room. Of course, the treatment wasn't long, and when I came out, to my surprise, all of my family was there! Needless to say, I was very emotional and surprised. So there everyone was—Bill, Buddy, Zachary, Jessica, my mom, dad, Joanne, Jaylyn, Dave and Grace. Brenda couldn't make it due to work, but they had her on the phone! Jessica had a flower and a certificate for me. I have to say she has the biggest heart for such a little girl. Remember the survey asking how I would like a celebration when I was done? Well Jessica was with me when I filled out the form, and I had put on there: "A flower and certificate would be nice." So she took it upon herself and got me those two things, AND she had the nurses sign it! I also had a basket of flowers that were sent to me, and everyone was waiting to see who they were from. When I opened the envelope, I was surprised to see that they were from Dr. H and staff. It was so nice of them to think of me.

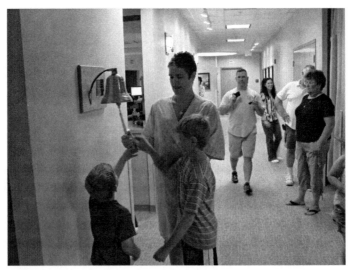

Zachary and Buddy helping me ring the bell to signify that I was done radiation treatments, Bill was taking the picture

I went down the hall and rang the bell and took a number of pictures. I was even touched to see that my dad had wiped a tear, but if you ask him, I am sure his eyes were just watering! Some of the nurses came and gave me hugs and told me that I have made them emotional and that it was so nice to have been able to meet me. I went to get dressed, and we all headed out of the building. But before we left, we took more pictures. This one we had to take because it was in the same spot as where we took a picture when I went for my consultation. You know, before and after. It will be good for the scrapbook that I will do, whenever that may be. Bill had to leave after ringing the bell but was very glad that he didn't miss any of the action.

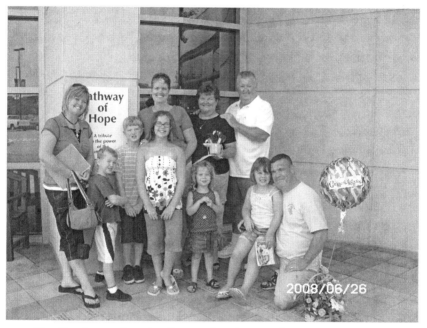

Family photo where it all started and now where it is completed

We headed to Brenda's for a birthday party for Grace. Buddy and I had to leave early for his all-star practice, but he was okay with that as long as Aunt Doe Doe brought him some cake. So it was a Thursday night, and I am all done with my treatments. Oh yeah, for those of you who sent me a charm for my bracelet—that I still don't know who started—you were all with me during my last treatment. I couldn't think of a better way to have all of your support, so if you missed saying hooray, you were still with me. Thank you again!

Friday, June 27, 2008

My first day without a doctor's visit. But I am still taking Zach to school, and I had to go to Dr. Hs to get my belongings. So I am still going into the direction as if I was getting treatment. UGH! When I got to the office, Deb was glad to see me, and we went looking for my things that were boxed up. It was very weird getting my things together, and my picture was still in my operatory. I feel bad for the girl who is replacing me because she had to look at me every day. Dr. H didn't ask me to come and get my things, but I feel as though they are taking up space. And even if I do come back, it will only be on Wednesdays, and I am sure not in "my" room. So why not go and get them. While I was there, Donna came up to see me. It was nice to catch up with her. Again, a bittersweet moment for me. I was so close to working there for fifteen years! I am going to miss my patients so much, but I know that this is the right thing for me to do.

Later that night, we headed to a Cub Scouts picnic. It rained but then cleared up, and we all had a good time. I received more congratulatory remarks on my completion. We got home, and as I was giving Buddy good-night kisses, he said to me, "Mommy, I am glad that you are done your treatments and that you didn't . . . you know, die." Well, if that didn't just touch my heart. I bent down and gave him the biggest kiss and hug and told him that I love him and that I am glad that I didn't die too.

Saturday, June 28, 2008

It still felt like a normal day because it was the weekend, and I didn't have any treatment today anyway. We did a service project at Connections Church called the Angel Food mission with the Cub Scouts, and they really enjoyed it, and so did I. I hope that we get to do it every month. I think the boys will get a better understanding by doing it more than once. We had lunch at the scoutmaster's house since there was leftover food from the picnic. We went home and had to get ready for Dave's welcome-home party. We could only stay for an hour because we had tickets for the Blue Rocks, and Bill was meeting us there. While at the party, many people came up to me and told me that I look very good and were very happy to hear that my treatment was done. We had a good time at Blue Rocks, and they actually won!

Sunday, June 29, 2008

Relax day. Not too much went on except getting ready for vacation! My skin is looking good. I have some peeling that is going on under my arm but not as painful. I am keeping the Aquaphor on it, and tonight, I am going to put some of the silver sulfa on it with a bandage. My energy level wasn't that low, but my daily twenty-minute nap came in handy.

Monday, June 30, 2008

I felt like I was forgetting something because guess what, I had no doctor's appointment, and I had nowhere to go! It is nice to be able to stay home and be "relaxed." The kids and I enjoyed the day, and they helped me clean so the house will be clean when we get back. It is the best feeling coming home to a clean house after vacation! Do I keep mentioning vacation to you? You can't tell that I am ready for it, can you?

Tuesday, July 1, 2008

I had an appointment with my therapist to go over bandaging. Buddy was with me and saw how it is done. It is more involving than I thought. It also amazed me that wrapping your fingers, hand, and arm will help lymphodema. Lisa told me that this is not going to stop swelling from happening, but if it does happen, I will know what to do.

We went over it a couple of times, and then I was on my way. Buddy and I got some Burger King and then headed to Payless for some sneakers. How bad did I feel when they sized his foot and his sneakers were almost two sizes too small! Anyway, we left there with seven pairs of shoes! BOGO is a good thing. We then went to K-Mart for some last-minute things for vacation and went to pick up Zachary from school. We aren't counting or anything but we only have two more days of day care!

Wednesday, July 2, 2008

Buddy had an appointment with Ms. Kym today, and I am happy to say that she felt he is doing really well, and we can come back on an as-needed basis. She said that during their session, they tried to play a game, and one of the activities was: Say something nice about your mom. His response was: "I am glad that my mom didn't die!" Obviously, that has been on his mind during this whole experience, but she said that it is very healthy for him to be able to express his feelings like that. So there is one more doctor's visit we can cross off our list! Bill and I went to our therapy session and it was a good one. We discussed where our life importance was prior to cancer and now after cancer. It was interesting to see how priorities change and to see how your partner changes as well. We had to fill out a survey, and home we went. When we got there Mom-mom was being covered with love from the boys, and I am sure that wouldn't be because she gave them money for vacation?

Thursday, July 3, 2008

I had an appointment with Dr. Warren, and even though I had to wait due to a delay in surgery, it was nice to see her. She was happy with my skin color and condition. She stated that it was not as "leathery" as it could have been from radiation. She is going to see me in about a month to re-evaluate me and talk about what my options are to start reconstruction. Again! We discussed about the bandaging that I was taught yesterday, and she recommended that I put it on prior to getting on the plane. This is not going to prevent it from happening, but it is going to start it working, prior to getting too swollen. So I guess I will be wrapping my arm in the airport. I don't want to do it prior to check-in because they will do a search on me because of the wrap. I don't need that, so I will wait. When I got home, I did last-minute packing, and the kids, Bill, and I are ready for vacation!

I will be sending you another update, but this time, it is going to be all about fun and relaxation. Believe me, I am not going to give you a day-by-day update, but I will fill you in on what we have done. Since this is on the laptop, which I am using instead of the hotel's, I can't or don't know how to get the pretty stationary or make it bigger, but I hope you enjoy the reading. And as always, I want to thank each and every one of you for praying for me, sending me cards, e-mailing me, calling me, visiting me, and just thinking about me. I have had a long journey and still continue that journey, but with the positive attitude and support from my family and friends, it hasn't been that bad. Not that I suggest it to anyone, but it is something that you can get through! I hope that you are enjoying your life and doing things you never thought that you would do. Thank you again, and I will talk to you again soon!

I'M BACK

Did you miss me? I can't believe that "summer" is over and that the kids are back to school. Boy, do I have some updates to give you. Don't get too scared, I am not going to give you a day-by day-outline. We'd be here for three days! Anyway, I do hope that all of you were able to enjoy your family and get some time away together. I certainly did. Okay, here we go with the update.

It is Friday, July 4, 2008 and the vacation got off to a great start. We took DE Express shuttle to make things easier for us. There is a lot of luggage when packing for thirteen days and four people. All went smoothly, and while we were waiting for the plane, I got all my goodies out to wrap my arm. It wasn't too bad, but it looked like I had a bad burn on my arm, and that is what the bandage was for. When we got on the plane and up in the air, a passenger didn't feel well. They asked for any medical personnel on board. Bill and another lady went up, and it was a lady whose son had the flu a couple of days ago and they thought that is what it was. The lady kept talking about food poisoning, but Bill seemed to disagree. The flight attendant came up to Bill later and thanked him again for his help. After talking to Bill, she asked if I was okay, looking at my arm. I explained what it was for, and she congratulated me. The rest of the flight went pretty quickly. We got our luggage and rental car (Chevy HHR) which was pretty nice. The room that we stayed in was only a one-bedroom room, but the kids enjoy sleeping on pull-out beds anyway. Remember when they used to be so comfortable? We thought that the tight quarters would be a problem, but it worked out fine. It forces you to be together and get along. After unpacking, we headed for the pool, which we did a lot of. Since it was July fourth, we went riding around to look for some fireworks sites, but the traffic was so bad we gave up and headed back to our room. This actually ended up being the better thing because we were on the seventh floor, and we could see fireworks from every direction, and we didn't have to deal with the traffic.

Two days into the vacation, my lovely red friend visited me! Doesn't it always happen that way while you are on vacation? I had prepared myself for the worst, but it actually didn't end up that bad. There were a couple of days, but nothing like that first episode. THANK GOODNESS!

We went to NASA on Tuesday, and the kids really enjoyed it. We saw a raccoon on the steps of the shuttle, which they found more fascinating. We were able to experience a launch, which was pretty neat. Zachary was only able to watch it on a TV screen because he was too short. Bill and I took turns. There were a little too many movies for the kids, but they enjoyed the touring of the launch pad and seeing a space shuttle up close. We went back to the resort and enjoyed more swimming.

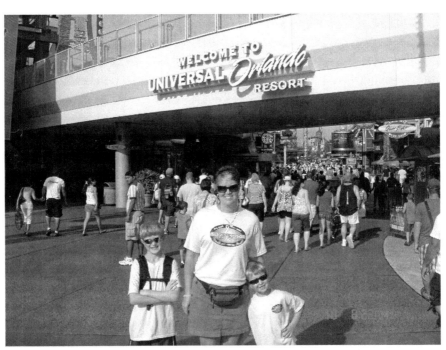

Buddy, myself and Zachary standing at Universal, Orlando, FL. Again, Bill is taking the picture

We did Universal, Islands of Adventure on Thursday, and the kids really enjoyed that. There were a couple of rides that they didn't do due to their age and height, but they said they liked it. Bill and I enjoyed it because it was not as crowded as Disney. We took a break in the middle of the day and went back to the resort. If anyone plans on going to a theme park, it is so nice taking a break in the middle of the day and then going back later on. You are refreshed and ready to go again. We enjoyed seeing the people who had been there all day and were not looking too happy. The break did real good for me. There was a lot of walking, but there were also plenty of benches to rest on. We had plenty of water too.

Saturday was for Downtown Disney, and we saw Cirque du Soleil. We really liked that. There isn't a bad seat in that place. We did some shopping prior to watching, and I will admit that this is one time when you miss having a girl with you. The princess area was so cool; there were little girls being made up to look like a princesses. I asked if the boys were interested, but they quickly said, "Ewww, no!"

On Sunday, we were back at Universal. This time it was Universal Studios. The kids enjoyed it there as well. They really liked eating at the Nascar restaurant. Our day was cut a little short because it looked like a storm was coming. When we got back to the resort, the sun was shining, and the pool was waiting.

We did the pool on Monday, and then went to Arabian nights. It was okay. Personally we liked Medieval Times better—more action. This was more about romance, but we had fun.

Tuesday was more pool time, but it was sort of a cloudy day. We didn't stay at Orange Lake where our time share was, but we did go and use their pools and amenities. We liked it there so much better. Later that night I started packing. It was a rainy night so why not pack.

By Wednesday, the kids were ready to come home. The weather was dreary, and I think they have had enough swimming. So we headed to Downtown Disney and did the Disney Quest for the day. This was five floors of video games and interactive activities. We all had a blast. We went back to the room to eat lunner (you know, lunch and dinner combined) and then headed back to Disney Quest. We were leaving the next day so we made the best of it.

Thursday, July 17, 2008, we were leaving and we were ready. In the past couple of days, the weather hasn't cooperated, and we have spent enough money. So needless to say, the plane was looking good. We left in the afternoon, which made it nice, and we could take our time. I prepped my arm again for the flight home. We had a nice flight and waited for our ride home.

———

So as you can see, we had a great time on vacation. I had a lot of relaxing time, and thank goodness for Bill because he hung out with the kids the majority of the time. I joined in some, but for the most part, I sat back and took it all in. I protected myself from the sun. Don't get me wrong, I do have a nice tan, but I was a good girl for my "treated" area. I didn't have to take any medicine for my throat, which by the way was all better by the end of vacation. The timing was perfect and well-needed. We all took some time to reconnect to the "real" life and enjoy each other. I also was able to finish a book while on vacation. Never would I think I'd be interested in Harry Potter books, but I couldn't stop reading it!

How quickly the craziness started back. Bill and I had our therapy session on Friday. It was okay, but we felt that they would help more if you do them while you are going through your treatment. It is hard to go back to what you were feeling. You would rather just move ahead, but that is why this is a study group for the HGC.

Saturday, July 19, 2008

It was Delaware City Day, and it was a HOT one. We got ready to see the parade, where, I might add, Dave was the Grand Marshall! After the parade, the kids went on some rides. I was not feeling too swell. I wanted to be back to normal so bad that I forgot it was still on the early side of that. I told Bill that I needed to go sit down in the shade and get some water. He got me something to eat as well, and I quickly felt better. Oops, I think I forgot to get something to eat for breakfast. Do you think that could have been it? Duh! Anyway, the rest of the day was great, and it was fun to be with family and friends.

During the rest of the month, we have been busy but with fun things. We went to the beach for the day with the kids. I met up with some friends for dinner. The subject came up about my prosthesis and how I did a show-and-tell at my son's school! Well, I didn't do a show-and-tell to the kids. It was to the teachers at Zachary's day care whom I know well, and the kids weren't around during that time. We laughed pretty good at that one. I went to dinner with my sisters, and how pathetic is this? We had to call our mom to ask where to go "hang out" for a drink! She came through for us too! My dad had some foot surgery and will not be able to put pressure on it for close to eight weeks! What will I do if I need him to be my chauffeur after my upcoming surgery?

Buddy's all-star team won! It was an awesome tournament. They were planning on going to regionals, but there was not enough players who could make it! We had to miss one of our therapy sessions, but it was totally worth it. Our group understood.

So this was an update on most of my summer. I figured I would update you on my fun stuff, and my next update will be for the medical side. You know how long they can be, and I don't want you to fall asleep reading them. So until tomorrow, I will talk to all of you then!

It Is The Medical Update

This is too funny! I couldn't send my last update because I had too many people on my list! I had to send it to two different groups!

Wednesday, July 30, 2008

I had an appointment with Dr. Biggs. I am happy to say that all is okay. There were no tests to be done just going by clinical signs. I did inform him that Bill was not too happy with that, and he explained to me again his reasoning. Some of you may agree, and some may disagree. Anyway, he stated that when I was diagnosed, we did the treatment necessary to remove the cancer (surgery, chemo, and radiation). There was nothing more to do to make sure that you get rid of it. That was the treatment. I can continue to go through testing, but that will make my life crazy! Say they see a spot on an X-ray. The only thing to do is to wait three months and test it again to see any change. If it is a false positive, I have spent the last three months worrying myself and OTHERS that I have cancer again. If the cancer comes back, most likely it is from the same cancer, and you then go from curing it to treating it. I am okay with that. I don't want to spend the rest of my life worrying and testing myself. As Dr. Biggs said, "Time is the best test anyone can have." He did mention to me that I could be a part of a study since I am premenopausal. There are three groups to the study: (1) continue taking Tamoxifen like I do now for five years; (2) continue to take Tamoxifen for five years but also suppress my ovaries from working by injection, radiation, or surgery; or (3) take a different drug (can't remember the name) for five years and also suppress the ovaries. You don't know what group you will be in until you sign up for the study. He gave me the information and took a blood test to check my estrogen levels. He told me to think about it and let

---

238

him know. I have thought about it and decided against it. Call me chicken, but if we know that Tamoxifen has been working, why change it? If I do get cancer again, I might blame it on being a part of the study, and to me, it is not worth it.

Monday, August 4, 2008

I had my checkup with Dr. Strasser. I took in some cookies for the gang to enjoy and to thank them for treating me. He was happy with the way the skin looks and pretty much says I am done! He will check me again in six months since Dr. Biggs is seeing me in three. Adios!

Tuesday, August 5, 2008

We had our last therapy session! We had to fill out a survey, and we got some of the group's contact information to keep in touch. After the session, there was a small group of us who talked about more personal things, which I wish we could have done at our regular sessions. But I know that the purpose of our sessions was not open forum. There was an agenda. Oh well, we met some nice couples and did learn some things about ourselves.

It is coming up on a year since I first felt the lump! Hard to believe, isn't it? August 7 was when I felt it, and August 9 was when I heard the dreaded word and had the biopsy. August 8 of this year, we went to the Blue Rocks sleepover with the Cub Scouts. The reason I brought up the year thing is that this time last year, we did the sleepover, and it was the day after my biopsy, so spirits are a little higher this year! We had a great time.

Monday, August 11, 2008

I had my appointment with Dr. Warren. She was also happy with the way the skin has healed and discussed my options. We didn't really discuss this one, but I could deflate the other side and have Brenda boobies (sorry Brenda!). The other two are ones that we talked about in the very beginning—the tram (using the belly fat and part of the muscle and tunneling it up to the breast) or the dorsal flap (taking a part of the muscle from my back and tunneling it to the breast and placing an expander). We went over the pros and cons, and I decided to go for the dorsal flap. The pro of the tram is that it uses your own tissue, and no expander is needed. The con is that it requires you to stay for four days in the hospital, and you need a six-week recovery. Also, there is an eight to ten percent chance that you could get a hernia. No, thank you! The way my luck has gone, I think

I will pass on that chance. Since part of the muscle is taken out, you are left with a whole. She explained that you know when you squeeze a balloon, and there is a weak spot and it pushes out? Well, that is what can happen to the stomach, and unfortunately there is not too much they can do about it. My luck. I would get a hernia and a "bubble." The dorsal flap pros are that it only requires you to stay overnight in the hospital, and it requires a three-week recovery. The con is that you still need to have the expander placed and go through the process of filling it and then having another small surgery for the transfer of the implants. I still feel that this is the better way to go for me and that both will look and feel the same—no comparison as to which looks better. So my surgery is scheduled Wednesday, September 10 in the Wilmington Hospital at 12:30 p.m. As I stated before, I will probably be down for about three weeks, so I am not going to be bashful and not ask for help. If anyone would like to drop off some meals, they would be greatly appreciated.

Later on, I had an appointment with my therapist. She just measured me to make sure that no lymphodema was going on. I had a little more swelling but not enough to have to do anything about. We will keep measuring and stretching. That is all that needs to happen.

August 15 to 17, 2008

We headed down to Chincoteague and had a great time. We spent the day at the beach on Saturday and had a campfire and headed home on Sunday. Nice and relaxing as usual. We wanted to have the last getaway before school starts on Wednesday!

Wednesday, August 20, 2008

Today was the kids' first day of school. Buddy was going into the third grade, and Zachary was going into kindergarten! They were both very excited for school. They woke up at three thirty in the morning, and I had to tell them it was still a couple of hours till school. They fell back to sleep and had no problem getting up in the morning. They were ready and at the bus stop twenty minutes early. I think that we are going to see a nice change with Buddy because now he is big man on campus, and he is taking care of his little brother. Joanne wanted to know if I cried when Zachary got on the bus, and I told her, "No, how could I, he was so excited and happy to go!" She said, "Yeah, but that is your baby getting on the bus!" I told her she would have my cry for me on her way to work. I also spoke to my boobie buddy, and she told me that she got emotional when her daughter got on the bus. Her thought process was that she was so happy to be there to see this happen! I didn't even think of it that way, and when she brought it to my attention, I was like *WOW, you're right. I'm glad that WE are here to remember this moment*!

My day was filled with servicemen coming in to check the maintenance of some of our electronics. So maybe tomorrow I will see what it is like with both kids on the bus and not having to drive to and from day care.

As I said before, I am happy to start getting my energy level back to where it was. I have tried to go for walks in the morning when the kids get on the bus. I am cleaning out some drawers and trying to keep up with cleaning the rest of the house. I am ready for my second haircut, and I believe that I am going to keep my hair short and not color it. I really like the quickness it takes to do my hair. As most of you remember, I am not that much of a hair or makeup person, so this suits me just fine. Buddy has started playing with my hair again. He says that he likes me better with hair, and it sometimes helps him to go to sleep. I have to say that I love it, and it relaxes me. I think that the kids are used to my hair, and they like me with the short hair. But sometimes, they don't like how it feels hard with the gel. Jaylyn continues to ask if my boo-boo is better, and I tell her it will be soon. The boys know and understand that Mommy is going in for surgery again to get a new boob! You gotta love it. Zachary is very affectionate and protective of me. If he sees Buddy or Daddy messing with me, he gets very defensive and sometimes upset that they are going to hurt me! It is so cute! I love them so much!

There is not too much going on the rest of the days prior to surgery. We will be having a family birthday day party for Buddy on Sunday. He is going to be nine years old! (The kids party is going to be on September 7.) We are finally changing his bedroom set. He has had the same one since he got out of the crib. I think he is due, and he has chosen the Phillies theme.

I will be getting measured again for any swelling on Tuesday. I will get my haircut on Wednesday. On Thursday, I am visiting my girlfriend whom I haven't seen in a while, and then I will meet with a dentist to talk about a job when I get finished with my recovery. I think it is going to be a good week. I will continue to read my Harry Potter book. I am happy to say I am on book number three, and I have gotten my Mom to read the first one.

I will continue to keep you posted on my progress and am glad to say that all looks and feels good. I am ready to get started on the "new" me. I remind you again to enjoy your life and what you have. Enjoy every minute

—

with your family, and let them know how much you care! Thank you again for the continued prayers for me and my family. I ask that you put in an additional prayer for my Aunt Sarah who is battling leukemia and lymphoma. She has had some pretty rough couple days and was put in the hospital. She is home now but is pretty weak. We will continue to be there for her and get every enjoyment of life that she has left!

My version of surgery

Monday, September 8, 2008

Two days before surgery! I had some errands to run and some cleaning to do. I stopped by Dr. Hazuda's to drop off my office key. I have to say it was like handing over your keys to your first house at settlement! I have been there since I graduated from hygiene school—fourteen and a half years ago. That's a long time. The girls were happy to see me, and I even got my teeth cleaned. She did a good job, but it definitely is going to be different for my patients/friends who were used to how I did it. I miss seeing my patients, and I hope they know it. When I got home, I started a little cleaning to prepare for my down time, but that didn't' last long because I have been starting dinner for the kids at around three in the afternoon so that it will be ready for them when they get off the bus at four in the afternoon. It has really worked out nice because they are starving when they get home, and they actually eat a good dinner as opposed to snacking when they get home and then not eating when it is dinnertime. This is one of the joys of being able to be home when your kids get off of the bus, and they appreciate it so much, more so the younger ones. I tell you this because so many of us get into the routine of work, work, work, and we don't realize how important it is to be there for our kids. I am speaking from experience, of course. Anyway, when I put the boys to bed, I talked to them about my surgery in a couple days and that I will be in the hospital overnight. Buddy wants to come and pick me up, but I told him that I will be home when he gets off of the bus. I think he is getting feelings of the cancer again because he asked how long the treatments would be. I reassured him that this surgery is not for the cancer because all that is gone and that I didn't need any more treatments. This is just so mommy can get her "new boobie." Zachary said, "Okay Mommy, so this means that I can only hug you around your waist, right?" They are so cute and understanding. We read some books like we always do, and off to bed they went.

Tuesday, September 9, 2008

I stayed home all day and got all of my cleaning and wash completed to prepare for my down time. It is like having a party at your house, and you want it to look spectacular! Remember how I just said it is good to be home for the kids when they get off of the bus? Well, here is another reason. Buddy walked in and had a different look on his face. I asked how his day was, and he said fine and then went straight to his room. Strange. My little guy said, "Mommy, Buddy got hurt on the bus today!"

"WHAT," I said and went back to his room. The door was locked, and he wouldn't let me in. I was in my room, and he opened the door. I asked him what happened. He looks as if he was about to cry and closed the door again. I told him that when he is ready to talk about it, I will be here to listen. Later on, he came out and told me that he and a boy got in trouble and will have to go to the principal tomorrow. Apparently, this boy started a comment that William pees the bed (unfortunately, he has a couple of times, and even though the kids on the bus don't know that, it still made him uncomfortable). The boy then punched Buddy, and he punched him back. And then the boy shoved Buddy's head in his book bag. Someone told the bus driver, and they both got in trouble. I think Buddy was more embarrassed than hurt. Anyway, we told him not to be afraid of telling the principal the truth, and it would be alright. I can't stand the bus! Not to mention that there are three people to a seat, and there is no kind of aide to watch the kids while the bus driver concentrates on the road. There is obviously going to be trouble. We'll see what happens tomorrow. But think about it, if I didn't get home until six in the evening like I normally did, he probably wouldn't have told me in that much detail. Who would have been there to help him through it like a mom or dad would?

We had a nice dinner. I filled Bill in on what happened, but all is okay now. I made sure I get a late snack since I can't eat after midnight.

Wednesday, September 10, 2008

Surgery day! We got the boys off to school and reassured Buddy that it would be okay. I didn't have to be at the hospital until ten thirty in the morning, but Bill and I had some errands to run before going there. Brenda called and asked me if I knew that my surgery was scheduled for 11:30 and not 12:30. No, I was told to be there at 10:30 for my surgery at 12:30. She said she was going to call and find out and call me back. Right before we left, she called back and said it was a false alarm and that the times are what I was told! We set off to run our errands. We arrived at the hospital at 10:20 a.m. I was having déjàvu, only this time I only had one boob walking in. I will say that last time, I was very glad that I worked up to the day before the surgery because I didn't really have time to think about it. This time, I felt like I was thinking more about it.

We checked in, signed the papers, and waited to be called back. As we were sitting there, Bill asked me why I told my family that they didn't have to be there. I got the feeling that he was getting flashbacks of before, and he was feeling a little nervous. I felt bad that he would be there by himself, but I think Joanne was planning on coming over for lunch. They called me back. I just sat there because I thought they said Mark not Hart. Oops! All the vitals were good. I got checked in, and they told me that I could go back out. They would call me back in about forty minutes. I didn't mind. I would rather sit out there with Bill than in the back. They finally called me back, and I got my pretty cap and gown on. They went to get Bill, and Brenda was with him (remember she works over at the surgicenter). I gave him a kiss and told him I would be alright and would see him in a little bit. They took my glasses, and I did the walk down the hallway, feeling blind. I told the nurse that Brenda works at the surgicenter, and she said that she could have come back, so where I had to walk, we saw Bill and Brenda again. Brenda grabbed my glasses and came back with me. It was so nice being able to see where I was going this time. Brenda had gotten a team together for me, and they were all SO nice. There were about four to five people who came in and were doing different things. They kept saying how happy I was!

Surgery update from Bill
Wednesday, September 10, 2008

> *Hey, everyone, it's Bill.*
> *I just wanted to let everyone know that it is now 12:07 pm, and Sharon is headed back to the room for her procedure. Keep your fingers crossed and the prayers coming, and everything will work*

out. I will TRY to put out another update later today; if not, I will do it tomorrow. I would like to thank each and everyone one of you for keeping her spirits up over the last year. It means a lot to both her and me.

Thanks again,
Bill

Here goes the IV, and of course, the only one that they could find was on my wrist (palm side). Yep, it's a sensitive one, but what are you going to do? Dr. Warren came in, put his initials on me, went over the process, and said we are ready. It is always a sense of relief when I see her. Brenda took my glasses, and I was off to the OR. Once I was in there, I scooted over to the OR bed. They were getting things ready. They put a mask over my face, and that is all she wrote. Next thing I remember is someone calling my name, and I felt pain and nauseated! They asked me how I was doing, and all I said was I felt pain and nauseated.

"Okay, we'll get something for that." As she walked away, I felt this overwhelming feeling of getting sick. You know how you start to swallow really exaggeratedly? I started taking deep breaths, and somehow, it did go away. Whether she gave me something, I don't remember. A little while later, they were wheeling me into my twenty-three-hour stay room. As they were wheeling me, they informed me that my family was at the end of the hall, so even though I couldn't see them, I waved to them so that I knew that they were there. Joanne told me I didn't look too sporty—pretty pale this time compared to last time.

Surgery update from Bill

Dr. Warren just came out and talked with me. I have not seen her yet, but the doctor said she is doing GREAT. She said that she smiled while going to sleep and smiled when she woke up. Sounds like she is still the Sharon we all know and love.

Thanks for all your support.

Bill

P.S. I am sitting here in the waiting room really close to Joanne and Brenda . . . LOL

They got to my room and asked me if I could walk to my bed. Are you serious? I don't even remember getting wheeled to my room. Somehow, I managed, and I did feel some pain. Once I got into my bed, the nurse (which is a male, Gerry) asked how I was feeling, and I said I was in pain. He said he would get some morphine to take care of it! Well, he stuck the needle in the IV, and OH MY GOSH, was that painful. I think he put it in there as fast as he could. It hurt so bad that I started crying. The next thing I heard them say was that they were going to go get my family. Oh great. I was sitting there, crying, and they were coming in. I tried to get myself together, but it didn't work. Then came Bill who went right to the top of the bed because he knew I was in pain. Then Brenda and Joanne came to the other side, asking what was wrong and what they could do. I finally got myself together, but it was just the pain from the medicine that he put in me. Afterwards, my vein got all swollen and red, which, they said, can happen with morphine (and I think on how fast you shoot it in a small vein. Duh!) They had another nurse (female) come in to check it. She aspirated some to make sure it was in the vein, and then put some saline in it. Ouch, ouch, ouch! Brenda asked if it could be changed, but the nurse said that it will be fine, and they will keep a check on it. Other than that, I did well. I reassured them that I would be okay. I think they looked at the surgical site, and we were amazed at how good it looked. But I can't remember too much. Brenda and Joanne left, and Bill stayed for a little while longer. He knew that I told him not to feel guilty about leaving me because Buddy had a ball game at night. We discussed this earlier in the week. So, he left, and I ate my ice and slept. They had these compression bags on my legs to prevent blood clots, a blood pressure cuff on, and my IV pole. Then I had to use the bathroom! I told the nurse and there I was, trying to get up. Oh yeah, there was pain. You can't believe how many different muscles you use to get up. Once I was up, I walked like an old lady. I made it to the bathroom and thought, *How do I do this? My left arm is sore from surgery, and my right arm has an IV needle in it at the wrist!* I managed to get my toilet paper before I sat down. Without being graphic, but you know me, as I wiped with my IV hand, I was thinking that the needle was going to come through the vein when I bend it! I managed, got up, washed my hands, and headed back to the room. They hooked me back up to everything, and I ate more ice. The funny thing about that whole IV is that the next day, Bill had filled me in that a needle is not left in my vein. It was just a little plastic "catheter" that was left there. We had a good laugh over that, but I wish I would have known that a long time ago. I have made it worse on myself!

Around nine in the evening, I talked to Bill and the boys, and while I was talking to them, Gerry came in to give me my antibiotic. I saw the needle and quickly told Bill that I have to go because I am about to get stuck again. When I got off the phone, I was all nervous for him to shoot it in me, but then he told me that it doesn't go in the IV where the morphine went in, it goes in up top and drips in. WHEW!, What a relief that was. In fact since then I have used the restroom, ate something, and my next pain medicine I can take in pill form! I called Bill and let him know that it was all okay, and we said our good nights. The night went by. I ate some saltines, read Harry Potter, slept some, watched TV, you know, the norm for hospital stay. Shift change. Yeah! I had two female nurses that time. I am not saying that male nurses are not good, they just don't have the care factor that women do unless they have female characteristics themselves. Susan told me that later on, we will be able to disconnect the IV and take it out!

Thursday, September 11, 2008
Surgery update from Bill

> *Sharon came home today and is resting at home. She is in a lot more pain with this surgery, but nothing that the pain meds can't handle. I am going to occupy the boys playing kickball and baseball for the next several days in the backyard to allow her some peace and quiet. Thanks for all your prayers.*
>
> *Bill*

The night went by. I felt like I got up a lot to use the bathroom. But this way, I got used to how to get up. The morning came, and my breath was nasty! They gave me a towel, washcloth, soap, toothpaste, toothbrush, and mouthwash. I immediately headed for the sink. It is amazing how refreshed you can feel just by washing your face and brushing your teeth. Don't be alarmed, I did bring my toothbrush, etc., but this came as a care pack. Oh yeah, and since my hair is short, I can even do that! My breakfast came, my first real meal since Tuesday, and it was good. The assistant, Ben, came in to check my surgical site. Now he knows his stuff and is very nice and cute too! He was very pleased with how everything looked and gave me my limitations—no lifting over three pounds, take it easy for the next couple days. He told me that the radiation really scarred me up and that I had a lot of scar tissues from that. They removed as much as they could, but there are limitations, of course. I thanked him so much for helping me out and hope that I don't have to come back there for that again. He agreed and said that I was "free to go." This was at nine in the morning! What happened to twenty-three hours? Man, they don't waste any time. I did tell them that Bill wasn't planning on picking me up until lunch time. They said that wouldn't be a problem. But I certainly saw a difference in the amount of times that they came to check in on me once I was "released." I was given my instructions again by the nurse. Bill got there around noon. He helped me get dressed. He went to get the car, and they wheeled me downstairs. The ride home was not bad, a little bumpy, but Bill did his best.

Once we got home, he had the couch all set up for me, but I chose to go back in the bedroom for. I slept while Bill went to get the Rxs filled. The boys came home and were happy to see me. Mom stopped by and stayed for awhile. She was amazed at how good the site looked. Dr. Warren was awesome! I am being faithful with my Percocet because if I don't, I get this knife-stabbing pain in my back! The front doesn't bother me at all. I had prepared myself that the donor site was going to be more painful.

I got through the night. Bill didn't sleep with me because he was so afraid of rolling over and touching the site. We had forgotten to empty my drains, so in the middle of the night, I went to bathroom and did that. But while I was up, I felt nauseated and finished up really quick, got the trash can, and laid back down. False alarm though, just a little hot spell. I took my Percocet and headed off to lah-lah-land.

As usual, I didn't leave much out. This is my update on the surgery, and I will give you a break here. My next update will be about my recovery.

Thank you again for all of your thoughts and prayers to help me get through this. It is hard to believe that a year has gone by!

More Recovery

Friday, September 12 to Sunday, September 14, 2008

If you remember, for my initial surgery, I had the Q-ball that released the anesthesia on a constant basis. Well, I had another one of those, but this time, it did not last as long. It was empty today, and Bill and I removed it. We were not afraid to do it this time.

Buddy had a baseball all-star banquet to go to on Friday night, and so that I was not by myself, we asked Mom and Dad if I could stay with them for the night. I ended up staying the whole weekend. I packed my bags, and Mom came over to pick me up. She felt much better that mommy was going to take care of her little girl again. I took my Percocet on a regular basis and I am trying to get used to getting up. It was still pretty painful when I try to get comfortable or try to get up from lying down. I got my rest and relax time in for the next couple of days. My drains continued to drain, but it was slowing down some. By Saturday night, I was noticing a very uncomfortable feeling in my back. I am not sure why I felt that, but when I lean back, I can feel the drain tubes moving. I can only explain it like this: you know how, say a tube lies in a track, and it may go off-track sometimes? That is what it feels like. It is not pain, just very, very icky feeling. Because of this, I am trying to move even less than before.

It was Sunday evening, and it was time for me to go home. Bill came to pick me up. I think he felt better that I was able to recover at my parents' instead of at home. Not that you don't want your kids around, but I was able to concentrate on recovery instead of attending to the kids.

Monday, September 15, 2008

My friend Amanda came over to stay with me in the morning and brought us dinner. She is a nurse practitioner, so it was nice talking with her. It also made Bill feel better because he was on day work, and he was so concerned with me being by myself. I am getting around fine. It just takes me a little while. I continue to take the Percocet and rest. Can you believe that I am doing what I am told and not doing anything! You know I have the temptation, but if I move the wrong way or use that muscle in the back, it is like getting a slash on the back of your hand. I rested in the afternoon, and the kids got home from school. They have been awesome, again, during this time. The weather was beautiful so their activeness could be released outside instead of inside. The drain tubes were still "jumping tracks," but I was getting used to it as much as I can and counting down for when they come out in eight days.

Tuesday, September 16, 2008

I rested all day and managed to go to Open House at the kids school with my mom that night. Bill took the boys to Cub Scouts. My mom thought that I was crazy for going, but I didn't want to miss it. Besides, I wouldn't be lifting or doing anything strenuous. The teachers were nice, and I hope for a good year.

Wednesday, September 17 to Monday, September 22, 2008

These days were pretty uneventful. Just popping Percocet, sleeping, and reading more Harry Potter. During the night, while changing positions or trying to get comfortable, the knife-stabbing feeling pain happens, but it is short-lived.

I had people stop by and bring meals and have lunch with me. Thank you, Kym, for coming more than one day and being "on-call" for me!

Tuesday, September 23, 2008

My sister-in-law, Cathy, drove me to Dr. Warren's. My dad was out of commission today due to his foot surgery. I felt anxious to get the drains out just because I know how my almost-fainting reaction was last time! I went back, and Cathy asked if I want her to come back, but I was more afraid of her passing out if she comes with me! Dr. Warren removed all of the tape that was on me, and I can't believe how great the incision site looked. She was happy with how the drains have slowed down and was ready to take them out. Ugh! She asked me if I was ready and continued to talk to me. One came out, and it wasn't too bad, and then the other came out. It is not a pain that you feel; it is just gross feeling something slide along the inside of your skin. Did you get the eebie-jeebies on that description? The next time I go to see her, she will start filling me again. When I left, I couldn't believe how awesome I felt! I was like a new person, but I know that I am still not allowed to be too active. I rested for the afternoon, and it felt so much better when I lean back. That night, Bill and I had a dinner that we had to go to for Zachary's preschool teacher whom we nominated for teacher of the year. It was nice to get out. She didn't win, but she did get recognized, and I think that meant a lot to her.

Wednesday, September 24 to Saturday, October 5, 2008

These days were spent getting stronger and starting back with some therapy two times a week. I have been moving around better and better each day. The kids continue to be active in fall baseball and Cub Scouts. They are doing well in school and seem to enjoy it. They sometimes forget about my incision areas but are apologetic when I kindly remind them that I am still not one hundred percent fine. So instead of playing kickball, I watch.

Monday, October 6, 2008

I had lunch with Angela. Remember the lady I reassured during her first chemo treatment? Well, we continued to keep in touch, and she was about to start her radiation, and I was reassuring her about that. She sounded so much more upbeat and positive. It was good to hear that.

Tuesday, October 7, 2008

I saw Dr. Warren for my first fill. Bill went with me. I am happy to say that due to my numbness, I didn't feel anything. She said that it went in very nicely. She put in sixty CC's! That is thirty more than what she would do each visit the first time. I will return in two weeks for another fill. Then, I needed to get home to get ready for my big first day at work! Yep, I am returning to work, but at a different office, of course. I had mixed feelings. I was ready to go back to the working world, but I was also going to miss not having any worries as to when to schedule or do things. I am starting back very part-time, like three hours a couple of days a week. I will eventually work every Monday and Thursday, but they are letting me work my way up to a full day. I spoke to the boys about going back to work, and I know that it will be an adjustment for them as well.

Wednesday, October 8, 2008

I got the boys off to school and went to therapy. I came home and got some lunch. Before I went to work, Bill got out the camera and said he needed to get a picture of me for my first day of work! He is so goofy, but I love him so much. So I got into my car, and in fifteen minutes, I was at my new work place. I will be seeing three patients because I am working from two to five in the afternoon. When I got there, the girls had a rose with a card in my room, and they had gotten a big chocolate chip cookie to welcome me to their office! I felt so welcomed! I was ready to start, but let me tell you, I am glad that my first day back is over. Not only being in a new office but not knowing the patients and trying to remember my routine was like seeing my first patient in hygiene school. I survived, and Dr. McAllister continues to work with me on my hours. Even though I continue to miss Dr. Hazuda's office, I still strongly believe that things happen for a reason, and that I was due for a change.

Friday, October 11, 2008

Bill and I had a special evening out. We went to the Hotel DuPont for the "Evening with Robin Roberts." She was a great speaker. We bought her book, got it signed, and took a picture with her. It was a nice night-out.

Sunday, October 12, 2008

There was a bunch of us, including Buddy, who did the "Making Strides against Breast Cancer" walk at the Wilmington Riverfront. It was a beautiful day, and we did do the lap two times. Some people only did it once. I was very happy to be there and able to walk it this year. I thank everyone who was there and supports the fight against cancer!

Monday, October 20, 2008

I had my final fill visit with Dr. Warren today. I believe that I had a second fill at some point, but can you believe that I don't remember when that was? I am happy to say that sixty CC's later, all is well! The incision sites are looking great, and I don't have much to report. I know that is unusual for me. She said that we are done with the fills and that we can schedule the

---

253

replacement. We just have to wait at least four weeks. I have to check my schedule since I work now (ha-ha). Before, I could just schedule. So I left there and shared the news with my family. I am almost there!

Tuesday, October 28, 2008

I have my sixth-month appointment with Dr. Biggs, and Bill went with me. He cleared me for another six months. YEAH! I also had Dr. Biggs reassure Bill. I had to explain to Dr. Biggs that I am not allowed to get sick or have any pain around Bill. He was at work, and I had told him that I had a stomach pain. He asked if I should call the doctor, but I tried to reassure him that it was just a gas pain. He asked how I knew, and I told him that once I released the gas, the pain went away! We of course laughed about it, but he just needed reassurance from the doctor. So Dr. Biggs explained that the only time that we need to let him know is when I have a pain that does not go away after one to two weeks or if I get a pain that goes away and then comes back and gets more painful. I think that this made Bill feel a little better. We will see.

So there it is! I am getting my life back to a normal state. I have scheduled my next and hopefully my last surgery for December 2! I am not going to remember what it feels like to have moveable boobies! It will only be a long weekend recovery. I will be sure to fill you in on the details.

As always, I share with you a little thought. Bill and I went to a Relay for Life University, and a gentleman made the comment that I have to agree with. He stated, "I am proud to say that I am a survivor and that recently I became a caregiver. I would have to say that if I had a choice to be a survivor or a caregiver, I would choose to be the survivor!" I strongly agree and understand that comment. If any of you have or are a caregiver you understand how hard it is to watch someone you love go through this process. You also know how hard it is to sit and not be able to take the pain away or do something about it. On the other hand, being the survivor, you can do something about it, and you know that it will be okay. So I applaud everyone who is or was a caregiver and thank you for what you have done! I continue to think positive, and nothing will stop me from living my life to the fullest. So, remember to have fun in your life and enjoy every minute that you have with your family.

On a sad note, I would like you to say a prayer for my family, especially my mom, who just lost her sister, my Aunt Sarah. She passed away Monday, October 27. She was battling leukemia/lymphoma, and even though she lost her battle, she won in my eyes. She was a very strong person, and nothing was going to bring her down. Even though she might have been in discomfort, she did not show it often. She fought having hospice come in, taking morphine, and getting a hospital bed in her home, as all of these things represented death to her. She did finally have hospice come in as I explained that they come to help you and that doesn't mean that you are going to die tomorrow. She was alert up to the last couple of days of her life because she didn't want to take the morphine. She knew that she would be able to spend as much time with her family as she could if she was coherent. As she finally had to take the morphine, she was in and out. As I visited her the day before she passed away, I will never forget that every time you would whisper in her ear, she would open her eyes and put on the biggest smile for you. As I was telling her how proud I was of her and how much I loved her, she managed to say, "No tears!" I assured her that I had none and told her to keep thinking happy thoughts. That night, the hospital bed came, and she passed away. So in my eyes, she won the battle that she knew she could handle. And that was when hospice came. But she didn't die the next day. She didn't take the morphine but for two to three days prior to her death, and she was only in the hospital bed for less than twenty-four hours! So you tell me who won in this battle? I love you Aunt Sarah, and will miss you very much!

TODAY IS THE BIG DAY!

Tuesday, December 2, 2008

I hope that you enjoyed your Thanksgiving with your family. I sure did and I actually tasted the Thanksgiving dinner this year. If you remember, last year, I was doing chemo, and my taste was all messed up. I am doing really well and feel great. I am working very part time but enjoy being in the environment and still having my family time.

The real reason that I wanted to e-mail you is that today is my big day! I finally get rid of my "turtle shells" and get my "marshmallows"! How exciting! This was the final surgery for me, and hopefully I will not have to make any visits to the operating room anytime soon. It is hard to believe how fast time flies, but we all got through this together, and I again thank all of you for your support, prayers, and cards. As you know by now, I will be sending you an update when I am done. I know that some of you may go through withdrawal from not hearing from me, and some of you may be glad. Either way, I am off to my big day. I have to be there by 10:30, but surgery isn't until 12:30. I am going to be so hungry, so enjoy your lunch for me!

Wednesday, December 3, 2008

Well, it is complete! The exchange was simple and quick. Bill and I got there at the Arsht Surgicenter and signed in, and they called me back, and I got prepped. One more wonderful IV. They were already starting to remember me. Not only because Brenda works there but also because of how hard a stick I am. Anyway, I gave my kisses to Bill, and he went out to wait. I got wheeled down (they have done this because I am so blind and they don't want me to run into anything) to the operating room. When I was in there, they asked me to climb onto the table, and they got things all ready. They showed me what the implants look like, and WOW, they look huge. Don't worry, I didn't go any bigger than I was prior to cancer. I will still be a nice C cup, but seeing it at this perspective, I would hate to see how big a D cup is. No wonder people with big breasts have bad backs.

I went to sleep, and when they woke me up, they informed me that all went well. They congratulated me. I am so happy that I don't have any drains any more. I got my post-op instructions. Dr. Warren said she wants to check me in two weeks and I was told to relax for a couple of days. When I got dressed, I was amazed that I only had a few steri-strips where the incisions were, and I was not feeling any discomfort. I haven't touched them yet. I think I was too scared right then. We drove home, and I relaxed for the rest of the day. In fact, I am resting today too.

Tuesday, December 16, 2008

I went to see Dr. Warren at 9:30, and she was very happy with the surgical site. She removed the steri-strips and the sutures and told me that she will see me in one month. She informed me that on the left side where they removed the lymph nodes and scar tissue, I have a "dip" in the under arm area. She did the best that she could to fill it, but that was the result. I also have to continue to be careful with shaving there as I do not have any feeling under there. When I return in one month, she said that we could talk about the final reconstruction of placing a nipple and tattooing the areola. This is an optional thing, and I don't know if I am even going to go that far. I have touched the "breasts," and it is funny how they are cold. I have not been wearing a bra, and Dr. Warren pretty much said that I don't have to anymore because that wearing bra is like a prop. Woohoo!

A Year in Review

Hello, everyone,

I was going through my updates, and I became very disappointed with myself. The last one that I have that I sent was dated December 16, 2008. If that was it, the only thing that I can say is that I am so sorry to have left you hanging like that. I am thinking that I am starting feeling so good and became so busy that I got sidetracked. So, what I have decided to do is to share with you a quick—yeah right—recap on my past year. I hope that all of you are doing well and that you enjoy this update. I will forewarn you that you may need to read it in a couple of sittings, but I want you to know just what I have been up to.

December '08

I lost a close friend, Michelle Smith, during this month. She was doing a cover-up with Wilmington Manor Fire Department, and she was hit by a car. Two days later, she passed away. It was a very tough time for many of us, and our thoughts are still with her family. It is coming up on a year, and I still can't believe that she is gone. We miss her smiling face so much. Rest in peace, Michelle!

Christmas was great; the kids totally enjoyed themselves, and I felt wonderful to be there healthy and happy.

New Year's Eve was celebrated at our house, and everyone enjoyed themselves. I of course was part of the entertainment because I found out a new trick that I can do with my right boob. When I tense up my muscle near there, my breast raises up. I did this by accident, and when I noticed it, it took me by surprise. I secretly showed it to my sisters, and they started laughing hysterically, which in turn led to having to inform everyone what we were laughing at. I can't do it with my left side, not yet anyway. I also celebrated my thirty-eighth birthday on that day!

January '09

We were, unfortunately, swamped with three funerals this month. They were all members of the firehouse. We were ready to start our year over!

I participated in the inaugural parade in Washington, DC on January 20 with the Delaware City Fire Company. It was freezing cold, and that day was very long, but I was glad I was a part of it. Funny thing, Bill participated in the inaugural events as well, but his was inside at one of the balls the night before the parade.

We celebrated Zachary's sixth birthday, and I can't believe how fast he is growing. We continued with scout activities, and we started planning for the Relay for Life, where we did another Beef-and-Beer. We also met with the principal of Southern Elementary and discussed having a mini Relay for Life at the school.

I had one doctor's appointment the whole month, and that was with Dr. Warren. Again, she was very pleased with the mobility. She said that due to the amount of scar tissue that the radiation created. She doesn't need to see me back for two months!

February

This month pretty much consisted of meetings for scouts, relay, school, and my Hygiene Association.

I only had one doctor's visit this month, and it was with Dr. Strasser, radiation oncologist. He was also pleased with the mobility. He said that most of the time, there isn't as much mobility at this early stage. He will see me in six months, which is halfway of my next appointment with Dr. Biggs. I am seeing one of them every three months.

March

We saw the Harlem Globetrotters and went snow-tubing this month. We all had a blast!

Had a number of meetings again but only one doctor's visit, and that was with Dr. Warren. We talked about the final reconstruction, nipple, and tattooing. I have decided not to do anything. I have gotten used to the way that it looks, and it doesn't bother me. My friend had the procedures done but was not all that pleased with it and had to have it redone. I can always change my mind in the future, but right now, I am keeping it plain. I will see her in three months.

I have decided to keep my hair short, and I continue to get compliments on it daily even with my gray patch of hair that I will not be coloring. So nice to pay less than $50 every six weeks!

Oh yeah, this was the month of Bill's surgery. Snip snip, if you know what I mean! Since I cannot take birth control any longer and we had already decided not to have any more children, we are playing it safe going this route. It was so simple. I can't believe more men don't help out their wives and do it. He was down for a couple of days, but it was pretty much an easy procedure.

April

We went away for a couple of days to CoCo Key Resorts in New Jersey. It was an indoor water park, and the kids had a blast. Two days of water fun!

Buddy was traveling with his baseball team, and he had his first tournament in Lake Shore, MD. His team came in second place, and that was because of loss of daylight and the absence of field lights.

Zachary had tubes put in his ears. There was no need for anything for his tonsils. He was looking forward to the surgery because of the ride in the wheelchair, the Icee's, and being off from school. He made out great!

I attended a Breast Cancer Emerging Hope luncheon where I saw a number of people whom I have met along the way during this journey. I also attended a seminar from Dr. Susan Love for the twelfth Annual Breast Cancer update. Dr. Biggs was a guest speaker at this seminar, and he had stated that there is a test that you can take that will tell you if Tamoxifen is working. I had a visit with him the following week, so I thought I would look into getting that done.

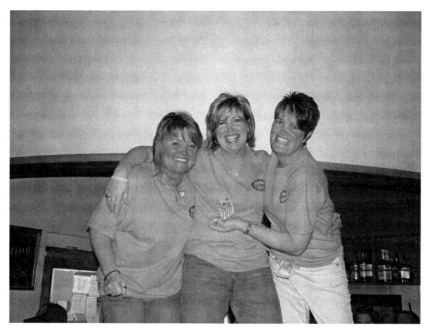

My sisters and I having fun on the bar at the
2nd Annual Team Survivor Beef and Beer

My big event was our second annual Beef-and-Beer for the Relay for Life team. We sold out on tickets, and it was a huge success. Bill played the video that he made about my journey and then it had clips from the relay from '08. It was very touching for a lot of people. We had a blast and look forward to April 30, 2010 for our next one!

May

One doctor's visit, and that was with Dr. Biggs. He gave me a six-month clear! Basically, I went in, and he examined me and sent me on my way for another six months. Some people may think he should have done more, but I am happy with it. I did ask him about these two spots that I have, one on each shoulder. They are red and flat, they do not bother me, but they have not gone away. He told me to put some hydrocortisone on them, and they should go away! I also asked about the test to see if Tamoxifen was working, and he said that yes, we could go ahead and get that done. He wrote me out a script for the blood work, and we went and I had that done. Later on, he called me while I was shopping, and Bill was waiting for me in the car. He called to say that the test results came back, and that I have what is called heterozygous. Something about one of my genes is defective, and that Tamoxifen is only working fifty percent. He went into more detail, but this is what I got out of our conversation. He explained that Tamoxifen works by encapsulating the genes to prevent any cancer to get to them, but since one of my genes is defective, it can't fully encapsulate it. He further explained that there really isn't anything that we can do for this condition. We don't increase the dosage as that won't do anything; there isn't another medication to use, since I am still premenopausal. So, we just continue to use Tamoxifen because at least it is working fifty percent. He mentioned that if I was to surgically put myself into menopause, then we can change to a different medication. But he doesn't feel that that is necessary. The news did not shock me because not too much has gone like a normal test, surgery, etc. would go. What I worry more about is how and if I tell anyone about this. I decide to keep this news to myself because there is nothing that we can do about it, and if I tell my family about this, then they will just worry themselves. But if in their mind they think that it is working one hundred percent, then that is less worrying for them. Which is when I also say to myself, before I took the test, I neglected to ask: What if the test comes back, and we find out that it is not working? If I never would have taken the test, I too would be thinking that it was working one hundred percent.

The next day, I informed my coworkers of the news and that I have chosen not to tell Bill or my family. All of them, especially Chrissy, felt that it was not a good idea. She lost her mother-in-law to breast cancer, and while she was living, she neglected to tell her son some important information about what was going on with her, and to this day he is upset about not knowing. She also put it in reverse. What if Bill had this information, and he did not tell me? I decided to tell Bill, but I was still not going to tell my family.

That night, we put the kids to bed, and I asked him if we could talk. I started off by saying, "Remember the other day when Dr. Biggs called?" Before I continued he said that he thinks he should sit down. I informed him about what Dr. Biggs told me, and his reaction was exactly what I had expected. He had the same look on his face as he did when I was told that I had cancer. I reassured him that it was all going to be okay. There is nothing that we can do about it, and we have to continue our lives as if it is working one hundred percent. I told him that I wasn't going to tell him, but thanks to Chrissy, I did. He told me to thank her for talking me into telling him, and we agreed not to tell the family for the same reason that I didn't want to tell him. It was a rough night for him, but we will get through this together. *(My family/friends will be reading this part for the first time, and I do hope that they understand why I kept it from them. But you'll see how things change for me later)*

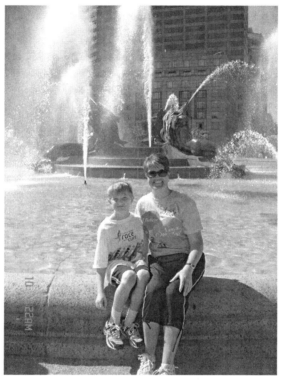

Buddy and I at the Susan G. Komen Race for a cure 5K in Philly.

On Mother's Day, Buddy went up with me to Philadelphia and did the Race for a Cure at five kilometers. We walked of course, but we had a great time and look forward to doing it next year.

Bill and I celebrated our thirteenth wedding anniversary! We also had many birthday celebrations this month!

Buddy had his second tournament at Ripken Stadium in Aberdeen, MD. It rained all day Saturday, but they still played and won. On Sunday, they played one game, and then the games were cancelled due to weather. His third and final tournament was in Washington Township, NJ. The kids didn't win, but they had a good time playing. Buddy was pitching and playing first base and left field.

I found out that a past coworker/friend of mine has breast cancer. She is in her thirties. I was in shock and have her on my mind constantly.

June

Bill and I put together a mini relay at Southern Elementary. Basically, the kids collected money in their classrooms for four weeks and raised over $1000! Each of the four weeks, they were given information about sun safety, tobacco, being fit, and eating healthy. On the Friday before the mini relay, we took an aerial picture with the kids spelling out the word HOPE. We were hoping to send this into the News Journal, but the principal that we have right now did not allow it. We were lucky that we were able to do what we did. On the actual relay day, we had honored the children who had or has someone who has been affected by cancer by giving them a pin with that person's name on it, and they wore a purple sash around them. They walked "the track," had water ice, did sidewalk chalk, bubbles, jump rope, danced, and had a great time! We also had requested that the kids dress in purple. We had an awesome response from the teachers and kids, but I am sure that we won't do it next year. It took a lot of planning, and we would rather do this with someone who feels it is just as important. I think it is a great way to educate children about cancer!

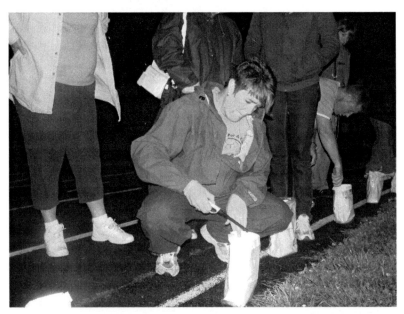

Me lighting my luminaria bag at the Middletown Relay For Life

June 5 was when the actual Relay for Life event was held. It rained this year, but it put no damper on the activities. I will say that it was more emotional for me this year than last year. I think that I was in my fight mode last year, and this year it all sank in what I had gone through the past year. We actually had three teams this year, and we plan on doing it again next year. So if any of you would like to donate or join our team, here is the website www.main.acsevents.org/goto/sharonhart. I am happy to say that we raised close to $13,000 this year.

I had a doctor's visit with Dr. Warren, and she checked out her work. All looked well with the implants/reconstruction. I showed her the two spots on my shoulder, and she wanted me to get them removed! She thought that they looked like skin cancer, and we would have them biopsied. I told her what Dr. Biggs told me to do and asked if she would send him a copy of the report. Isn't that interesting? I guess oncologists only deal with "inside-the-body" cancer. Anyway, she just told me to keep them covered in the sun, and we scheduled it for July 8th. I think this would be the easiest procedure for me so far.

Buddy, Zachary, Mom, Joanne, Jessica, Jaylyn, and myself went on a vacation to Massanutten. This is near the Shenandoah Valley. Bill had to work and couldn't take another week off, so I asked if he minded that I take Mom and Joanne. Of course, he wished he could go, but was okay with us going and just wanted us to have fun. Well, that we did. The kids did plenty of swimming, putt-putt golf, go-kart riding, and looking at all of the deer. My mom stayed back at the room for most of the swimming part, but we felt like we had a maid service. The wash was done, the beds were made, and dinner was ready. We felt bad, but she kept telling us that she was fine and that was what she wanted to do. We also visited the Luray Caverns, which everyone really enjoyed. Oh yeah, and while we were at a water park, it was towards the end of the day, and I was lying there when saw something on the inside of my left arm. I went to wipe it off, and it didn't move. When I looked again I noticed it was a very small tick! I quickly scratched it off, and then realized that part of it was in my skin. As I was trying to pick it out, I was sitting there thinking, *Oh great, it is a deer tick, and it is in my left arm; and now I will probably get Lyme's disease!* The kids were in the water, so they didn't know what was happening, but I did go to the lifeguard to get some tweezers. Well, if that wasn't a joke. The tweezers were plastic and all bent at the tip, so they sent me to their first-aid room. This was another joke. It was this young guy who acted like he was scared of me. He told me that he was unsure what kind of tick it was since it was only the remnants that he could see. He wasn't allowed to use these other tweezers to get it out. So I asked him if I could do it! I took them and was determined to get this piece out. It finally came out, and he opened the cortisone and Band-aid but didn't apply it. It was very weird, but all was well, and then I basically just had to wait if a ring appears or symptoms occur. This did not put a damper on the vacation at all. Besides, we only had one more day before we left. We had many laughs, and it was a great time being together! Oh yeah, and so I don't leave you hanging on this part, there was no ring that occurred and no symptoms. Yeah!

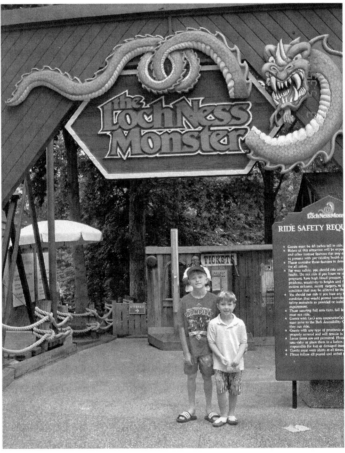

Buddy and Zachary in front of their first roller coaster,
"The Lochness Monster" at Busch Gardens, Williamsburg, VA

Buddy had Cub Scout camp the next week, and the following week Bill, Buddy, Zachary, and I went to Williamsburg for the week. We had another awesome time, and this was the kids' first time to get on roller coasters. They loved it! I think Bill was more excited about it than they were. We went on the Loch Ness Monster ride five times! I was nervous because of Zachary, but he loved it. He was so excited that he was tall enough to go on other rides. It was a moment to remember. Wow, they are getting so big!

We also went to Water Country, USA, and I think we went on every ride. It is a great park to go to, not too big.

I felt good during the whole time and was glad to have my health back this year. We stayed covered in sunscreen, and it was so easy to get the kids to put it on.

July

On July 8, I had my surgery to remove the two spots on my shoulders. I had it at the surgicenter at Glasgow since it was just local. They were very nice there, and I even saw one of my patients from Dr. Hazuda's. The surgicenter has individual rooms where you are in while you are waiting. Nice privacy. The surgery went great. We talked during the whole procedure. I didn't really feel anything but the needle to get numb.

I saw her again the following week for a follow-up, and the test results showed that it was in fact skin cancer but not the kind that will go internally. In fact, she said that it is not about whether I will get another spot but rather when. So she said that when she sees me in six months, we would do a body check for any suspicious areas.

The rest of the month was filled with day camps for the kids, meetings, doctor's appointments for the kids (who are healthy), work, and baseball games. Buddy made the all-star-team for Bear Babe Ruth, and they won. So we would be going to Troy, NY for the regional tournament.

August

Beginning of August, we went to Troy, NY for the regional tournament. The kids played great, but unfortunately were beat in the end. It was a great experience for them all.

We did the sleepover at the Blue Rocks again with the Cub Scouts. I was in charge of getting this together for our pack. Not a lot of planning. The fun thing was that Zachary was a Tiger Cub Scout this year, so he was actually included. Bill was going to take off for this, but the boys said it was okay if he saved the vacation for another day.

School started on August 19. Buddy is in fourth grade, and Zachary is in first grade. Yikes! We are looking forward to a great year.

I had an appointment with Dianne, the nurse practitioner at my OB/Gyn. I told her about some occasional discomfort that I was having in the lower abdomen area. Due to my history and it being so hard to detect ovarian cancer, she decided to order an ultrasound to check things out. She was not concerned but wanted to be on the safe side.

So the next day, I get my ultrasound, and they found a cyst on my ovary. Dianne sent me a letter and wanted me to get another ultrasound in two months to recheck things.

Buddy turned ten on the thirty-first, and we had his party at the Christiana Skating rink. It amazed me how that place has not changed since I used to go there.

September

Scouts were in full force, but we had two of them in it and two different groups. So it was challenging.

This month, we planned a sleepover at Brenda's house—just the sisters—to hang out. As I have always said before, it is so important to spend time with your family, and this was great for us to reconnect. I will never take for granted the relationship that my family has!

My mom and dad celebrated their forty-fifth wedding anniversary, and we went to the Cowtown Rodeo to celebrate! We actually didn't go because of that, but it happened to be on their actual anniversary date.

We went camping with two of my friends Merith and Melissa and their families. We had been planning this for so long, and of course, it rained that weekend. Friday was a washout, but it didn't stop us. We decided to have a sleepover at Merith's house. The kids were even-numbered and played great together. The adults played board games and had just as much fun. We got up in the morning and headed to the campsite. The rain had stopped, and it was just an occasional mist. We had a blast and can't wait to do it again. So, as I say how important family is, friends are just as important!

I had my check-up appointment with Dr. Strasser. He did a look/see, and there were no concerns. Another six-month clear! I am not sure how long I will be seeing him, but to me, he is just another doctor to keep his eye on me.

I was in a golf "tournament" with the firehouse. My team was with three other ladies, one of whom was my mom. Like myself, she has never played real golf before. We had practiced a couple of times at Vandergrift, but we definitely are far from pros. The "tournament" was really just to get the ladies auxiliaries together and have a good time. Well, that we did. We named ourselves the "Golden Golfer," and Bill and my Dad were our "Golden Caddies."

That Saturday, was the Firemen's Conference, and I was actually able to be in the parade. The past two years, I was out because of surgery, so I was looking forward to this year. Buddy was on our Fire Prevention float, and Zachary chose to stay at Joanne's. Bill had to work.

October

No doctor's visits this month. Buddy did get high fever and headache for three days. Who knows if it was part of the swine or not, but he was down for a couple of days. All was well.

Middle of the month, we had the Webelo Wood's weekend campout. All four of us were going to go, but it was a rainy mess. So Bill and Zachary came down Friday night to help us set up. And then they went home. Zachary was supposed to have a ball game the next day, and Bill was taking him. So I had suggested that they just help us set up and then go back home. My thinking this way was because it was very muddy, and with four people in a tent and one of them being six years old, it would not be good. I didn't know that I was going to hurt my husband's feelings by telling him to go home. Heck, if I would have known that, I would have had him stay; and I would have gone home because I have never seen so much rain. Buddy and I hung in there and stayed the whole weekend minus the rain. The boys had a good time and did well.

I was planning on doing the three-day walk, but I didn't have enough time to train or raise the $2300 that one has to raise. Maybe next year or the year after that. LOL.

My friend who had breast cancer was doing very well. She had a double mastectomy and reconstruction, but thank goodness she did not need to go through chemo or radiation. She is in remission and enjoying her life in a whole new aspect.

November

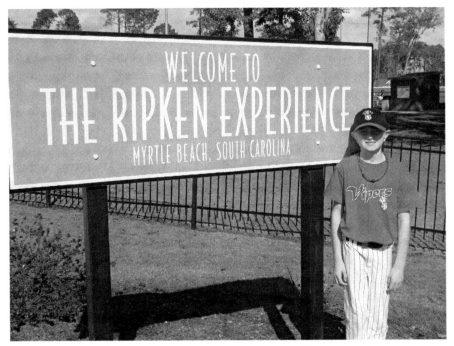

Buddy at the Cal Ripken Experience in Myrtle Beach,
South Carolina

Buddy continued to travel with his baseball team. This month, we had a tournament in Myrtle Beach, North Carolina. We left Friday, October 30, and came home Monday, November 2. Zachary stayed home with Joanne so that he could go trick-or-treating. He first wanted to go with us, and then as time got closer, he decided to stay. So, my mom decided to join us. We had a really good time. The boys did not play their best, but they had a good time together. I was glad that my mom joined us so that she could see how Buddy has come along in baseball. I think Buddy really enjoyed it as well.

I had another sixth-month check up with Dr. Biggs. Besides waiting for fifty minutes before being seen, with no magazines or radio playing in the exam room, all was well. He did an over-all check and ordered some blood tests to check my levels. I have been having some dizziness and headaches, but he was not concerned about that. He again tried to reassure us that if a symptom occurs, goes away, and then comes back, and it is stronger, then we need to let him know. Since this is something that has only happened recently, he wanted me to keep a watch on it. Bill didn't like it at all but would accept it then. I informed him of the cyst that they found, and we discussed taking the ovaries out. But he did not feel that was necessary right then. He said we had to see what the next ultrasound would show since cysts are very common.

All of my blood work came out normal. So we were cleared for another six months. I did have to ask Bill why he wasn't happy when we left, and he said that it was because he worries about it happening all over again. I asked him to be happy in the "now" and enjoy what we have. As I have said before, you can't control the future, so you have to take it as it comes.

We stayed overnight on the USS Constellation in Baltimore, Maryland with the Cub Scouts. This was another thing that I was in charge of. Bill does not like it when I am in charge of these things. He feels it takes too much of my time and takes time away from him and the kids. I feel differently, but you can't always agree on everything. The kids had a great time, and we learned that sleeping on a hammock with a sleeping bag does NOT work out that well.

I had my second ultrasound done, and it showed that I have three cysts. I didn't go into a panic about the news but more for what or if I would tell my family. I went straight over to Terranova's office, and she told me that she wanted to talk things over with the doctor. She ordered a blood test—CA 125 I think is the name of it. She didn't really like this test because if I have any kind of other infection going on, it may come back with a high number unrelated to the cyst. Basically, if this test comes back with a high number, it could mean cancer. I questioned her about just taking the ovaries out and being done with it. She told me that it was an option but not to jump to anything drastic. I called Bill and told him about the results. I also told him not to worry, but I could tell that he was so worried and was getting that same feeling all over again. That afternoon, I had lunch with Joanne, and she asked how things went. As I was not able to lie, I told her what was going on. She was nauseated but kept saying that she was trying to be like me and think positive. Then, Brenda called, and I filled her in on what was going on. She is the one who, I know, will take it like me.

Later that day, I had an appointment with Dr. O'Neill. I have had continued headaches and some dizziness. They were not getting worse, but I noticed that they were happening. He was not concerned with the symptoms either. He did an exam on me and said that we should just keep a check on it, but again he was not concerned. Basically, Bill was a nervous wreck that

I could have brain cancer and couldn't understand why Dr. O'Neill didn't order an MRI or a CAT scan to check things out. Bill didn't express this while we were in the office because he said he would have gotten nasty and said things he shouldn't. While I was there, he strongly suggested that I get a pneumonia shot, so I did as he suggested. I have already got the H1N1 shot. I also filled him in on what was going on with the cysts, and he informed me that doing the hysterectomy is not an easy surgery. I have to consider the hormone change, hot flashes, etc. that I may have. Before I jump to the extreme, see what the biopsy tells and go from there.

A couple of days passed, and Terranova called me and told me that my test levels look great. She wanted to schedule a look-see/biopsy and go from there. What I have found out is that women always have cysts from our menstrual period, and even though I have not had a period since May, I am still premenopausal and somewhere/somehow having a menstrual period. I am a little confused, but I will not complain that I don't have that mess once a month. So, I had a procedure scheduled for January 8. I questioned the length of time before the procedure, but it was another two months down the road, and we could still see if more will have appeared. They didn't say that, but it sounded good to me. They just said that it was okay to wait.

I think I now know why I was getting headaches and dizziness. I was getting sick! I was down for three days with a high fever and a headache, so I guess I can knock out brain cancer. Oh, I am sorry, I know that some of you didn't find that funny, but you have to remember our saying—to cope is to joke!

Remember my friend Michele Smith who was killed in the line of duty? Well, the verdict came in, and the suspect was found guilty on five counts! This means that at the least, he will get life in prison. Of course, there will be an appeal, but the sentencing is scheduled on January 2010. So we continue to pray that justice is served.

On a sad note, a lady (she was in her forties, and you never know how to address women that age) whom I knew lost her battle with breast cancer on Thanksgiving night. Each time I hear of it, it affects me more and more. She had two children—teenagers—and a husband. It, again, puts life into perspective and makes me realize how important it is to enjoy every moment we have. I look at my kids, and I love them so much. I look at my husband, and I love him so much. I look at my family, and I love them so much. I enjoy every waking moment, and I try to live life to the fullest. So, as you have read this long book of mine, you can see that I am not stopping.

Some people think that I push myself too much, but there will come a time when I can't do these things. But I won't regret any activity/event that I have done! I love my life!

December

I had a doctor's appointment with Dr. Warren. All was fine, and she will see me in six months. These visits are getting easy.

This month, we were busy getting ready for the holidays. No need to go in to detail as to ALL of the events I have done. Since you have been reading this update for an hour already, I will give you this Christmas present and just tell you that I am so appreciative of all that I have. I am thankful for my family, friends, and my health. I continue to thank all of you for listening to me while I went through my journey. I couldn't have done it without you. I apologize again for not updating you after my last procedure, but as you can see, I went right into active mode and have been very busy.

I continued to keep my hair short, and I loved it. I continued to get those black hairs on my chin and looked like a Chia Pet at times. My nails have gone back to normal. There was still numbness in my right big toe. I don't have to wear a bra, but I will say I now understand why men get that sweat line underneath their chest and women don't. Women wear bras, and it collects there!

I continued to work two and a half days a week and volunteered at the boys' school as much as I could. Bill and I would go on lunch dates whenever possible, and we continued to be very happy and in love with each other. My boys are my life, and I love every bit of my time with them. Darla, well, let's just say she loves me very much. If you want to ever visit me, just watch your ankles, she may try to taste them. She is so cute though that you can't help but love her.

That was my year in review. I will try to inform you of what goes on in January, but I am not getting worried. And you shouldn't either. That especially goes for you, Mom! I wish all of you a very happy holiday season and a healthy New Year. Enjoy every minute of your life, and don't forget, DON'T SWEAT THE SMALL STUFF! Now, go out and have a snowball fight or build a snowman with your children or significant other!

Happy New Year!

I thought that I would give you a quick update on my surgery. Well, I haven't had it yet! I had an appointment with my Ob/Gyn, and we decided to go for the partial hysterectomy. She told me that she was going to just take out the ovary with the cysts on it and that if I wanted to, she could take the other one out at the same time. Through discussion, we agreed to schedule to do this. This will reduce the risk of reoccurrence. Bill and I are not planning on having any more kids. My fear is how I will handle menopause, but I know that I will get through it. This also means that I will be changing my Tamoxifen to probably Arimidex, but I will wait to hear from Dr. Biggs about that.

Anyway, I changed the date of the surgery because we had a skiing trip planned last week, and I wouldn't have been able to go if I had the surgery on the eighth. I will be down for about a week. My new surgery date is scheduled for Friday, January 29, so I will let you know how it all goes.

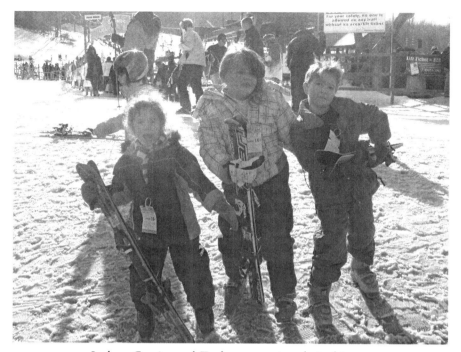

Jaylyn, Gracie, and Zachary sporting their ski gear
at Shawnee Mountain

I was able to go skiing, and we all had a blast. I was with my family—Joanne, Jessica, Jaylyn, Brenda, Dave, and Gracie. It was all of the kids' first time to ski. There were tears for some, but we were very proud that they did it. Buddy was moved up in his class for doing so well, and he was able to go down some blue squares with us. Zachary was like a white streak going down the mountain. He had no fear, and he did not quite know how to turn or slow down. But as the day went on, he did better. Jessica was able to go down a number of times. She conquered her fear. Jaylyn and Gracie, well let's just say they had their skis on. This was another moment where I have to say how great it is to have such a great family. We all enjoyed being together, and my sisters and I had some quality time together. I hope that all of you can try to schedule this with your family and enjoy yourself.

Happy snow!

I couldn't wait to send you this update, and since we have twenty-four inches and more of snow, and we are in a state of emergency, what else is there to do?

Friday, January 29, 2010

It was the day of the surgery, and Joanne met Bill and me at the surgicenter after she put the kids on the bus. I gave the kids hugs and kisses and told them to have a great day and that I should be home by the time they get home from school. Bill and I headed on our way. As I was checking in, I saw a past patient of mine. She was glad to see me and heard that I am doing well. After we checked in/registered, we headed to the waiting room to sit. This was my first time at the Christiana Surgicenter so I didn't know how they work there. But Brenda did have a team all waiting for me. They called me back, and I asked the nurse when Bill would be able to come back. She told me that I would see him after surgery.

"What?"

She said that it is because of that "wonderful" HIPAA rule stating that they can't come back and wait with us. So I went out and told him that I love him and gave him a kiss. I didn't get to see Joanne before I went back. It was the second time that she has missed me going back, but she did call and tell us that the bus picked up late, and that was why she was not there yet. Anyway, I was taken to the bathroom. The nurse handed me the bag of clothes to change into, asked me some questions, and told me to come out when I am done. Before I came out, I took the arnica that my sister's friend had given me to prevent bruising. I took it prior to my mastectomy.

I don't know if it worked, but I was doing it again. The only thing was I can't remember how much I am supposed to take, and I didn't get in touch with Brenda to ask. So I took three pills and put them under my tongue to dissolve. I headed out, and the nurse took me into this little room to go over my surgery, take my vitals, and eventually get the IV placed. Since it was not time for the surgery and I had to sit there, I asked her if she could get my book from Bill. I have been reading "My Sister's Keeper." My niece Jessica gave it to me for my birthday, and we were having a race to see who could finish it first. She was winning right now. It is a great book!

The anesthesiologist came in, went over some things, and then looked for the vein. He found one in the hand, and I started asking my questions. I thought that the needle actually stayed in, but he was showing me how the needle comes out and how it actually has a little "umbrella" on it that covers the needle when it is pulled out. Pretty neat stuff if you don't get woozy about things like that. He told me that they were not quite ready for me, but he took me into this waiting room where there were other patients waiting to be taken back for procedures. While I was waiting, the "team" that Brenda had set up for me came out and talked to me. I have met them before but couldn't really remember them with all of their gear on. I felt kind of like a celebrity with all of the special attention.

They finally were ready for me. They took my glasses and book and put them in my locker. I told the nurse that I was going to have to hold her arm as I am practically blind without my glasses. She took me into the cold operating room, and everyone was waiting for me. I was introduced to some of the other team members, and they got me all situated. Dr. Schubert came in. They apologized for her not being able to talk to me prior to getting me back, she and wanted to know if I had any questions. I said that I would take their word for it that it was her because I couldn't see anything and definitely couldn't recognize her with her gear on. They said that they have to go over a couple of things prior to getting started. The nurse took a hold of one arm, and Dr. Schubert took a hold of my other arm. They just stood there. I thought to myself, *Are they about to pray or what?* Then they started laughing. The anesthetist forgot that she was the one to start, and all it was, was to review what was being done to me and to see if I was ready. They put the mask on me and told me to take a couple of deep breaths, and out I went.

Next thing I remember is them waking me up, and I was in another room. They told me that they were about to take me into the post-op room to sit for a little bit. I needed to get up into this chair, and they reclined it and rolled me into another room. They closed the curtain and told me that they were going to go and get Bill and Joanne. I was feeling pretty good, just very dry and cold. They got me some hot tea and some graham crackers. Yum yum, not! Bill and Joanne came back and were happy to see me smiling as usual. The nurse came in again, took out my IV, and went over some instructions with us. She told me that I could get dressed and that Bill could go and get the car. Wow, I felt like I was being thrown out of there. I mean, I just woke up. Couldn't they give me a little more time? Bill got the car, and Joanne stayed with me. I stuck out my foot, and Joanne said, "What, you want me to put your socks on for you?"

"Uh, yeah," I said, and we started laughing. I asked for some water before I left and made sure that they passed on the message that I really thank the team for being with me today since I didn't get a chance to say it in the OR.

I got into another wheelchair, and they started to wheel me out. Joanne asked me if I was feeling fine because I looked really pale. I told her that I am okay. I got situated in the car, and we remembered to take a bed pillow with us to put in between the seat belt and my belly. (This is always a good tip to remember) We headed home, and on the way, I got this really nauseous feeling and got really hot, but I closed my eyes, asked to have the heat turned down, and relaxed myself. I made it home, but I think Bill was pretty worried that I was going to get sick in the car, so he drove a little faster than the speed limit. I don't remember everything either since I probably still had drugs in me.

When we got to the house, my mom was there waiting for the kids. They had a half-day, and we weren't sure if we would be home in enough time. As I was walking in, I said a few words, but then I started to feel nauseated again. I went straight back to my bedroom and lay down. Much better. In fact, I didn't even change out of my comfy clothes. There wasn't much pain, but I could feel it when I had to get up. The kids came home and ran right back to see me and make sure that I was okay. They gave me kisses and headed back out. I took some catnaps but got woken up by them a number of times. I didn't get mad because I knew that it was because they were worried about me and just wanted to make sure that I was okay. Bill made a couple of phone calls to get my follow-up appointment and also to Dr. Biggs to check and see what I was supposed to do about taking Tamoxifen. They informed him that I would need to start taking Arimidex and that they would call in the prescription for me. We were surprised that they didn't call us prior to the surgery to go over that with us. I will bring this up the next time I see him. *(This is what I meant when I said things would be changing for me. I can now let my family know about the Tamoxifen only working 50 percent, I hope that I saved them nine months of worrying. Again, my point with everything happens for a reason.)* It came time for my nieces to come home from school, and they couldn't wait to see me. Jaylyn made me a card and a heart and gave me a plastic ring to wear.

Bill sent out an e-mail to my family and friends to update them on my surgery. This is what he sent out to everyone:

January 29, 2010

Hey everyone it is Bill.

Sharon wanted me to let everyone know that she is home from surgery and doing well. The dr. said when she in there she did find another cyst on her right ovary as well. Sharon had already planned to have this one removed. After surgery the dr. told us that all the cysts looked like normal cysts. She did not see anything suspicious with them just by looking at them. She will still send them out for a biopsy to verify that they were benign and we will get the results in a couple of weeks. LET'S KEEP OUR FINGERS CROSSED.

She is now up in bed just relaxing. I think she deserves a nice rest and it is well-deserved. I would like to personally thank each and everyone one of you for your continued support since her diagnosis in 2007. It means a lot to me, and I know how much it means to her. Thanks for being there for us . . . You never know the true meaning of a friend until something like this happens, and now we know the true meaning.

Remember to do self-exams . . . It could save your life . . .

Thanks again for everything

Bill Hart

Bill went to get my prescription, and Mom had put on a crock-pot of meatballs and sauce for dinner. We all ate when he got back, but I was told not to eat any acidic foods. So I just had plain spaghetti with butter and cheese. I didn't stay up too long. Back to bed I went. The night ended with my mom bringing over a snuggie that she had made out of the breast cancer ribbon fabric. It is so soft and long, with a pocket for my feet. She ended up taking Jaylyn and Zachary to her house for the night. Bill hung out with Buddy while Jessica stayed with me in bed. We watched the movie "My Sister's Keeper." You talk about a tearjerker of a movie. We couldn't even talk to each other; we were crying so hard. It had a great message, and after we calmed ourselves down, we talked about it. She ended up staying with me for the night, and Bill slept with Buddy. It was another one of those bonding moments that are priceless. I continued to take my Vicodin for the pain, and it seemed to have kept it at a minimum.

It was a good day, and the surgery went well. I will say that now that I have tried the three surgicenters (Arsht, Glasgow, and Christiana), I liked Christiana the least. Everyone was nice, but there is not much privacy, and it doesn't seem as personable for that reason. I don't have any complaints, but I just thought that I was not kept there long enough after I woke up. What is the medical system coming to?

I spent the following days spent lying in bed. I actually did nothing but take some pain meds for a couple of days, and then I rested, watched television, and read. Bill took very good care of me during that time, and I surprised everyone by actually doing nothing. By Wednesday, I was feeling better, but then I have gotten a nice head cold, sneezing (which is not fun right after surgery), headache, and runny nose.

Friday, February 5, 2010

We were suppose to get a snowstorm later in the day. Bill went to work for night shift, and they told him to come prepared to stay until Sunday morning because of the snow. It started snowing around four thirty in the afternoon and didn't stop until late the next day. We got twenty-seven inches!

Sunday, February 7, 2010

Bill finally got home in the morning and used my brother-in-law's tractor to plow off the driveway. Then he was bedbound. I felt very good, and I love snow. I couldn't stand not to go outside, and since I felt really good, I decided to go and shovel. I knew I had to take it easy, and it was light snow. Bill did the majority of the work, and I just shoveled a path to the front door. The sun was shining nicely and melting it off of the driveway. I spent a good part of the day outside, and I felt good. I didn't think that my mom agreed with me doing it, but I know my body, and I am very much like my dad with lifting the proper way.

Good News Tuesday!

Tuesday, February 9, 2010

Today is what we call Good News Tuesday. I had my visit with the doctor today to get the results of the biopsy. It was snowy, but the main roads were pretty clear. My mom came over to watch the kids since school was closed due to the snow. When we got there, they told us that Dr. Schubert was out sick but that they didn't want to cancel our appointment. This made me nervous, thinking that they didn't want me to wait because it was bad news. We were sitting there, waiting, and the other doctor came in, went over how the doctor wasn't there, and apologized. Meanwhile, Bill and I were like "Okay, okay, just give us the results." Well, we are happy to say that the results say that it is a normal benign cyst. Big sigh of relief from the both of us. He checked the surgical sites and said that everything looks to be healing well and that my only limitation is not to lift more than twenty-five pounds. I told him that I shoveled, and he said that was okay. He wants me to be careful with lifting because I am still healing on the inside. We left, and I made the phone calls and sent out the text to my friends that it is good news.

I will continue to take Arimidex instead of Tamoxifen. I will continue to take calcium supplements and have my recall appointments with Dr. Biggs, Dr. Strasser, and Dr. Warren. I hope no other events happen, but if they do, I know for a fact that I can handle whatever comes my way! Positive thinking is a powerful thing, and I am proud to say that I have that quality! The one thing that I am waiting for now is good old menopause. My mom tells me not to worry because I will probably go through it being even happier than I already am. I can only hope.

—

MY FINAL THOUGHTS ABOUT MY JOURNEY!

I personally want to thank all of you again for being there with me during this journey. I hope that I have helped you to understand what cancer is all about and that you can get through just about anything. Family, friends, and prayers are such an important thing to have in your life. Without them, one can find themselves struggling. You can try to find the good in almost anything. Life is a wonderful thing, and I hope that all of you will remember these things:

1. Live life to the fullest.
2. Don't sweat the small stuff.
3. Don't put off the things that you want to do; you may not get to do them.
4. "To cope is to joke."
5. Finally and most importantly, love your family and be thankful for what you have!

Love to you all, and thank you again for your support during my journey, now go check your breasts!

Sharon

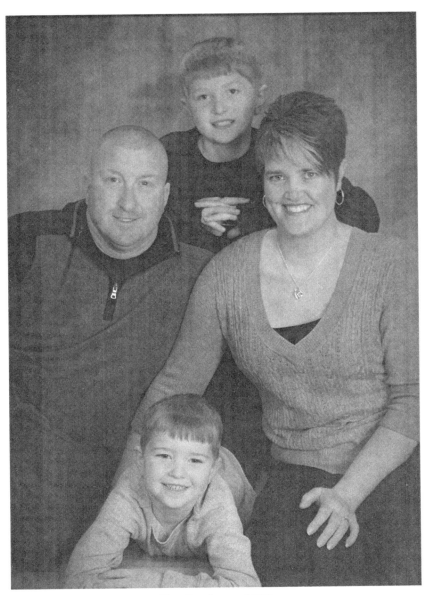

Family photo, 2009

Breinigsville, PA USA
16 May 2010

238075BV00001B/5/P